ACCLAIM FOR

WHAT YOUR DOCTOR MAY NOT TELL YOU ABOUT™ IBS

"I wholeheartedly endorse Dr. Ash's natural, commonsense approach to the pervasive problem of IBS."

—Ronald Hoffman, M.D., author of *7 Weeks to a Settled Stomach* and past president, The American College for the Advancement of Medicine (ACAM)

"This book is for the many people who suffer with IBS day after day, year after year, without any help beyond drugs that give them unpleasant side effects. . . . This book advances our understanding of how our bodies work and of how we can achieve lasting, robust health."

—John Parks Trowbridge, M.D., author of *The Yeast Syndrome*

"Dr. Ash has succeeded in transforming a bewildering and complex subject into a highly understandable and rational presentation. . . . An elegant and articulate presentation of the subject that should become a first-read by any physician or patient interested in improving this debilitating condition."

—Philip Lee Miller, M.D., founder and director, Los Gatos Longevity Institute

"Using his own experience as a guideline, Dr. Ash has developed a drug-free program using natural remedies. . . . Readers of this book—follow his advice. I can assure you, it makes all the difference in the world—it works."

—Jason Binn, publisher of *Gotham, Hamptons,* and *L.A. Confidential* magazines.

What Your Doctor May *Not* Tell You About™ IBS

Eliminate Your Symptoms and Live a Pain-Free, Drug-Free Life

RICHARD N. ASH, M.D.
with WINIFRED CONKLING

A Lynn Sonberg Book

WELLNESS CENTRAL

NEW YORK BOSTON

This book is not intended to treat illness or replace consultation with a medical professional. If you have symptoms of irritable bowel syndrome or another gastrointestinal problem, consult a physician with expertise in digestive disorders. If you are currently on prescription medication, consult your doctor before discontinuing it or taking supplements of any kind.

Wellness Central
Hachette Book Group
237 Park Avenue
New York, NY 10017

www.HachetteBookGroup.com

Warner Wellness is an imprint of Grand Central Publishing.
The Wellness Central name and logo are trademarks of Hachette Book Group, Inc.

Printed in the United States of America

First Edition: June 2004

10 9 8 7 6 5

Library of Congress Cataloging-in-Publication Data
Ash, Richard N.
What your doctor may not tell you about IBS : eliminate your symptoms and live a pain-free, drug-free life / Richard Ash, with Winifred Conkling.
p. cm.
Includes bibliographical references and index.
ISBN 978-0-446-69091-1
1. Irritable colon—Popular works. 2. Irritable colon—Alternative treatment—Popular works. I. Conkling, Winifred. II. Title.
RC862.I77A84 2004
616.3'42—dc22 2003015967

Cover design by Diane Luger
Book design by Charles A. Sutherland

To my wife, Dorothy Ash,
who has always been my inspiration and life partner.

Contents

Introduction ix

Chapter 1 Why a Holistic Approach Works When Traditional Medicine Fails 1

Chapter 2 Your Digestive System and IBS 9

Chapter 3 Do You Have IBS? 24

Chapter 4 Understanding Food Sensitivities and Food Allergies 45

Chapter 5 Living with Milk Intolerance 55

Chapter 6 Candidiasis, or Yeast Overgrowth 64

Chapter 7 How to Customize Your Diet to Beat IBS 75

Chapter 8 Meal Plans and Recipes to Make Eating Right Easier 97

Chapter 9 Relax Your Mind, Relax Your Colon 117

Chapter 10	Exercise for a Healthy Body and Healthy Bowel	136
Chapter 11	Nutritional Supplements	152
Chapter 12	Putting It All Together: Thirty Days to a Healthier Digestive System	166
Chapter 13	Gluten Intolerance (Celiac Disease)	195
Chapter 14	When It Isn't IBS: Understanding Other Digestive Disorders	207
Conclusion		221
Resources		223
Index		230

Introduction

Most people who walk into my office complaining of diarrhea, constipation, cramps, and other digestive problems feel that they are alone in the world. They often feel embarrassed to discuss their symptoms, seeking help only as a last resort. In truth, an estimated one out of every three Americans regularly battles digestive problems, such as irritable bowel syndrome (IBS).

IBS sufferers typically turn first to the corner drugstore or pharmacy for help, where they pick up over-the-counter laxatives, antacids, fiber supplements, and antidiarrheals. They spend more than $3 billion on these nonprescription products, hoping for a cure, but almost never finding one.

That's because the conventional method of treating IBS does not work. In my experience, most of the products commonly used to treat IBS actually make the problem worse. To treat your IBS and eliminate your symptoms once and for all, you need to look at your body holistically. I did not reach this conclusion by chance; it took years for me to appreciate the need for a more comprehensive approach to medicine and healing.

When I started practicing medicine as an internist in 1979, I practiced conventional medicine. I would examine a patient, find out what was wrong, label the condition, and reflexively prescribe the most current drug to alleviate the patient's symptoms. As time went on, I noticed that instead of getting better, most of my patients returned needing higher doses or stronger medicines. I don't want to disparage drugs; they are essential in the treatment of acute illness (such as a heart attack or pneumonia), but their record is much less impressive in the treatment of many chronic illnesses (such as arthritis or allergies). When it comes to treating ongoing medical problems, such as irritable bowel syndrome, medication is not the answer. In these cases, medicines end up masking the patient's symptoms, when what the doctor needs to do is to determine the cause of the problem.

I changed my medical philosophy in 1985 when I was diagnosed with severe joint pain and a form of arthritis called gout. I consulted various experts, all of whom recommended drugs to reduce the inflammation. Over time, my pain became more frequent, and I required higher doses of stronger drugs. At one point, I was taking the maximum allowable doses of the powerful anti-inflammatory drug prednisone, and I had cortisone injected into my joints.

I questioned this approach, but I did not suggest any alternative treatments. As a doctor, I knew the high risk of gastrointestinal bleeding and immune system dysfunction, which can be caused by excessive use of anti-inflammatory drugs. As a patient, I experienced fluid retention, stomach upset, weight gain, cataracts, and thinning bones caused by the long-term drug therapy. In addition, I learned that the medication was inhibiting my adrenal gland, breaking down muscle and protein, and causing high blood pressure. Every time I tried to lower the dosages of the drugs I was taking, my symptoms returned with a vengeance. Despite my side effects, the traditional medical establishment had no other treatments to offer me.

This medication-based approach was the standard of care recommended by the leading doctors in the field, and I followed it for more than two and a half years. I was in pain; I wanted relief. Like many other patients, I felt I had few other choices.

Despite the high doses of various medications, my pain continued. I went to yet another rheumatologist, an expert in joint pain, who prescribed allopurinol, a drug to lower my uric acid levels. After three days on the medication at one-third the prescribed dose, I had blood in my urine, abdominal pain, and high blood pressure. The doctor conducted various blood tests, which revealed a dangerously low blood platelet count—a condition known as thrombocytopenia—as well as elevated liver function tests, which showed early signs of liver damage caused by an allergic or hypersensitivity reaction to the medication I was taking. What had started as joint pain resulted in a systemic breakdown that nearly cost me my life. If I had continued to take the allopurinol, I have no doubt that I would have died.

During the course of my illness, I saw eight different doctors at eight leading medical institutions, and they all recommended the same treatment. I now understand that I was looking for a sunset in the east; I was looking for a cure in an arena where a cure does not exist. I had exhausted all conventional treatments, and my condition had done nothing but deteriorate.

I realized that I had to approach my healing in a new way. I gave up on traditional medicine and began to treat my condition holistically. I read journals and attended conferences on alternative medicine. I worked with several specialists at the National Institutes of Health; I identified various foods and chemical sensitivities; specifically, I learned I was hypersensitive to sodium benzoate, a preservative commonly used in processed foods, and vinyl chloride, a contaminant in our water supply. (The PVC tubing in my water filter system contributed to my exposure.) I also found I was sensitive to organic carrot juice, which I had been consuming in large quantities, assuming that such a nutritious food would be good for me.

I knew the medications I was taking could do nothing but mask my symptoms, so I began to lower the doses—gradually, since I suffered rebound attacks each time I took less medication. It took six to eight months to wean myself from the prednisone and anti-inflammatory drugs I had been taking. I was able to make these changes only after I had begun to use various alternative treatments that alkalinized my body.

This experience both eliminated my joint pain and changed the way I practice medicine. My experience taught me that most chronic illnesses are more effectively treated if you identify the source of the problem and treat the cause, rather than work to eliminate the symptoms. This approach is particularly effective in the treatment of irritable bowel syndrome. This book is designed to help you identify the root cause of your digestive problems, so that you can heal your digestive system without masking symptoms or relying on medications.

USING THIS BOOK

While no book can replace a hands-on, face-to-face meeting with an informed physician, in this book I present the same information I would give you if you came to my office at the Ash Center for Comprehensive Medicine in New York City. If you follow the advice in this book, you can begin to improve your IBS within thirty days, even if you have spent years going from one doctor to another.

Most books on irritable bowel syndrome offer advice on how to minimize symptoms; this book strives to help you discover the cause of your bowel problems so that you can bring your system back into balance. I will help you understand how to alter your lifestyle to strengthen your gastrointestinal system and improve your quality of life. The traditional diagnose-and-medicate approach to treating IBS can actually alter the pH of the gastrointestinal tract, interfering with overall digestion. Not only can this traditional approach lead to a variety of side effects, but it can also aggravate gastrointestinal problems.

Even if you slept through high-school biology, if you suffer from IBS you probably have developed a renewed interest in understanding your digestive system. While chapter 1 outlines my overall approach, chapter 2 defines irritable bowel syndrome and offers a primer on how a healthy digestive system works. Chapter 3 helps you determine whether you suffer from IBS, and it describes the tests that might be used to diagnose IBS as well as other digestive disorders. This chapter will demystify the diagnostic medical tests that doctors typically use, and it will explain several tests that most traditional doctors do not perform, though they provide essential information about digestive health.

Food sensitivities trigger many episodes of IBS. Chapter 4 clarifies the differences between food allergies and sensitivities, as well as the differences between immediate and delayed food reactions. Chapter 5 describes lactose intolerance—sensitivity to milk and other dairy products—which tends to afflict most people with IBS. Candidiasis, or the overgrowth of yeast, is another digestive system imbalance that can be fueled by poor food choices and by the use of conventional medications used to treat IBS. Chapter 6 describes the yeast syndrome and offers specific information on how to change your diet and lifestyle to get your yeast levels back in balance.

Many people with IBS fear food and are painfully aware that the wrong choice at the dinner table may lead to hours of agony in the bathroom. Chapter 7 provides detailed recommendations on which foods to eat—and which to avoid—to keep your digestive system at peace. Chapter 8 offers meal plans and some recipes to make cooking easier.

Emotional stress can trigger IBS symptoms. Chapter 9 demonstrates the mind–body link between emotions and digestion, and provides information on how to control your bowels by controlling your emotions. Regular exercise also has been found to help relieve IBS symptoms; chapter 10 reviews the importance of exercise to bowel function and provides information on how to start a simple exercise program, regardless of your current state of fitness.

In addition to avoiding the wrong foods, you must also provide your body with the nutrients it needs to rebuild. Chapter 11 describes the vitamins, minerals, and other supplements that can be used to bolster the digestive system.

Chapter 12, "Putting It All Together," helps synthesize the information provided in the book. It includes a day-by-day plan description to help you put the information you have learned into practice. By following the prescriptive advice offered in this chapter, you can enjoy improved digestive health within thirty days.

It must be noted that the symptoms of IBS can resemble those of other digestive problems that do not respond to the advice I give for treating IBS. Chapter 13, "Gluten Intolerance (Celiac Disease)," describes this potentially disabling condition. If you have celiac disease, you need to be under the treatment of a medical professional with alternative medicine experience or a qualified nutritionist. Chapter 14 describes other digestive disorders that sometimes resemble IBS. It is important to recognize the symptoms of other digestive disorders so that you can seek appropriate medical care.

Many people spend years going from doctor to doctor, searching for an explanation of their gastrointestinal woes, without ever finding satisfaction. Prevention is preferable to treatment, and the only way to prevent chronic illness is to regain systemic balance throughout your body. It is my belief that by following the advice in this book and searching for the underlying cause of your digestive distress, you can overcome IBS and live symptom-free.

WHAT YOUR DOCTOR MAY *NOT* TELL YOU ABOUT™

IBS

Chapter 1

Why a Holistic Approach Works When Traditional Medicine Fails

A thirty-two-year-old woman came to my office complaining of all the classic symptoms of irritable bowel syndrome (IBS): heartburn, abdominal cramps, bloating, and alternating bouts of diarrhea and constipation. She had been to a gastroenterologist, who conducted several tests to determine that she did not have an ulcer; he then prescribed Zantac, a popular prescription antacid.

After several days on the drug, the woman felt much better. Then a new set of symptoms appeared. She developed a white tongue and rectal itching (signs of yeast overgrowth), and she suffered from pain on the right side of her rib cage (a symptom of liver inflammation). She told her doctor about the symptoms and he switched her to another prescription antacid.

Months went by, but the woman's side effects never subsided. She then heard me speak on the radio about IBS. She made an appointment and came in to see me, explaining that she felt I had described her situation exactly on my radio show. After a series of diagnostic tests, I found that her sensitivity to dairy products was off the charts. I asked her about her eating habits, and she told me she ate a "healthy" diet, except for the six or seven cups of coffee she drank every day, supplemented with cream and sugar.

Everything her doctor had told her to do was making her situation worse. Her doctor never discussed the importance of changing her diet and testing to see if she was milk intolerant. He never told her to limit caffeine intake (which exacerbates IBS) or to restrict her sugar intake (which feeds the yeast overgrowth that had occurred as a side effect of the drugs she was taking). In fact, the antacids the doctors had prescribed altered the pH in her digestive tract, actually making her symptoms worse.

This woman ate foods that were so irritating to her digestive system that they were almost the equivalent of eating glass. She wore her body down by consuming allergenic foods and taking the wrong medications; she failed to build her body up by consuming the vitamins, minerals, and nutrients her body needed. The more food she ate that acted like glass, the more inflammation existed in her gastrointestinal tract and the harder her body had to work to repair the damage. At some point, she ate so much "glass" that her digestive system was unable to stay ahead of the repairs. She developed persistent inflammation and IBS.

At my recommendation, the woman eliminated dairy from her diet, avoided trigger foods that contributed to her IBS, took various vitamins to decrease inflammation in her gastrointestinal tract and to balance her bacterial flora, and stopped taking the prescription antacids. Within two weeks, she felt much better. By the end of the month, she felt better than she had in years.

This woman's story mirrors those of many of my patients with IBS who are failed by traditional medicine. These patients first turn to prescription medicines for relief of their symptoms. The medications may provide temporary relief, but in time the symptoms—or new ones—will reappear. They eventually ask for help in detecting the root cause of their discomfort. Once the imbalance in their digestive system is corrected, they can experience normal bowel function again.

A NEW APPROACH TO HEALING

Philosophers say that the eyes are the windows of the soul; I believe that the gastrointestinal tract is the window to overall health. Our GI tract has two functions: It allows the body to obtain nutrients from food, and it keeps toxins away from the body. We have a finite amount of energy or reserve capacity to fight toxins in the environment, to manage the physical and emotional consequences of stress, to compensate for vitamin and mineral deficiencies, and to combat food sensitivities. When the body is overstressed, the digestive system tends to be the first to break down—and one of the first warning signs of digestive imbalance are the symptoms of IBS.

Most people have experienced this phenomenon firsthand. From time to time, we all suffer from the pain and humiliation of digestive distress. For most of us, these unpleasant symptoms pass in a day or two, but for the forty million Americans with IBS, diarrhea, constipation, bloating, and cramping are a fact of life. The condition is not life threatening, but it can compromise quality of life as sufferers stay at home to avoid painful episodes in public places or at work.

Except for the common cold, IBS accounts for more work

and school absences than any other illness. Americans spend more than $3 billion a year on over-the-counter medications to manage digestive problems, and billions more on prescription medications. While these medications may relieve symptoms for a brief period of time, they do nothing to treat the cause of the digestive problem. Your doctor probably has not told you how to manage IBS without turning to over-the-counter and prescription medications to control the symptoms. There is a new paradigm in the treatment of IBS: We can and must deal with the problem, rather than suppressing the symptoms. This is the crux of the holistic approach.

Despite the logic of this approach, some patients approach alternative therapies with a great deal of skepticism. I usually ask them about their history with traditional medicine, which typically involves a series of misdiagnoses and medications, none of which solved the problems. Then I tell them to remember a time when they searched for a missing item, such as lost car keys. They may have opened the kitchen drawer and looked for the keys, but found nothing. They may have thought some more, then checked the drawer again, tearing through old papers and sighing heavily. They may open the same drawer six or seven times, without realizing that looking almost anywhere else is a better choice than looking in the same drawer again. Too many people continue to come back to the drawer of conventional medicine to cure their ills, even when they don't find what they are looking for there. At some point, the only rational decision a person can make is to open up to other possibilities. Often people must become distraught before they open up to new choices; they must experience frustration with conventional medicine before they can consider other treatment options.

HOW MOST DOCTORS GET IT WRONG

For most patients with IBS, conventional medicine will never provide a lasting cure for their condition. With some medications, the symptoms of IBS may subside temporarily, but in time they often reoccur—and sometimes with a vengeance. In my experience, there are seven common problems with the traditional approach to treating IBS:

Problem 1: *Most doctors treat the symptoms of IBS, rather than searching for the cause of the problem.* IBS is a description of a group of symptoms; it is a label of exclusion, not a diagnosis of a specific disease. IBS is a sign that the digestive system is out of balance. When dealing with a patient with IBS, most doctors turn to drugs before doing the detective work necessary to determine the cause of the digestive disturbance. I use medication as a last resort, not the first choice of treatment. Rather than masking the symptoms, a doctor should find out what is irritating the digestive system and eliminate the cause.

Problem 2: *Traditional treatments will actually make IBS worse.* When facing a patient with IBS, most doctors reach for a pen and write a prescription for Tagamet, Zantac, Pepcid, Prilosec, and other drugs to inhibit the release of hydrochloric acid in the stomach. The optimal pH range in the stomach is 1.5 to 2.5, with hydrochloric acid being the primary stomach acid. The use of antacids raises the pH above 3.5, which inhibits the acid in the stomach that is responsible for the digestion of proteins. This change in pH also alters the microbial environment throughout the digestive tract, weakening the "good" flora and encouraging the overgrowth of "bad" flora.

The patient may feel better temporarily, but the digestive problems will become worse over time. These so-called cures actually exacerbate the digestive imbalances that caused the problems in the first place. Many people with heartburn and IBS need additional stomach acid, rather than the elimination or neutralization of stomach acid.

Problem 3: *Medications used by traditional doctors often have unwanted side effects.* Popular drugs used to treat IBS are far from benign. They often may cause yeast and digestive flora imbalances, which can further stress the digestive system and contribute to immune system suppression. Instead of using prescription drugs, I recommend the use of vitamins and nutrients to heal the digestive system—and, of course, the patient must discover which foods are stressing the digestive system.

Problem 4: *Most doctors dismiss food allergies and hypersensitivities as irrelevant, although they are a major trigger in many cases of IBS.* Most gastroenterologists believe that diet does not affect IBS; there is no doubt that it does. While some doctors begrudgingly acknowledge that lactose intolerance can cause digestive problems, they fail to appreciate the significance of other dietary factors as a trigger for IBS.

Problem 5: *Most doctors use IBS as a catchall diagnosis when they have done an upper GI series, colonoscopy, and endoscopy, and they see inflammation or gastritis but do not know the cause.* IBS is not a disease; it is a collection of symptoms indicating that the body is out of harmony. As an approach to treatment, most doctors perform several tests to rule out ulcers, cancer, infection, and other common disorders, offering diagnosis by exclusion. Patients need a diagnosis and a prescription, so doctors label them IBS patients and order up prescription-strength antacids. Instead, a doctor should work with the patient and perform the necessary diagnostic tests to determine the actual cause of the digestive complaints. Diagnostic tests are available that can measure the antibody response to certain foods. These tests should be a standard part of the treatment of IBS, but few doctors are aware of their value or recommend them.

Problem 6: *Most doctors are satisfied before their patients are cured.* A majority of doctors assume their patients have been well treated when their symptoms subside, even if they later return. The doctors' goal should be the elimination of the cause of irritation. It's like prescribing morphine to someone in pain because he or she has a nail in their foot. Morphine does not treat or cure the nail; it only eliminates pain. Doctors need to find the nail and take it out in order to solve the problem. The doctor's job is not done until the root cause has been identified and balance has been restored to the patient's digestive system.

Problem 7: *Most doctors fail to recognize the importance of environmental factors in triggering IBS.* Psychological and lifestyle factors also contribute to IBS. These issues must be dealt with head-on, rather than setting them aside in favor of reliance on medication. A growing body of research indicates that psychological stress triggers IBS in many people, and that many relaxation techniques can be effective in controlling stress—and IBS.

While the conventional approach to treating IBS fails in many ways, the information presented in this book will guide you through a new approach to treatment. You will learn how to identify the foods that cause digestive distress and how to nourish your body with vitamins and supplements that will help you rebuild your digestive system. Even if you have been suffering with IBS for years, the material presented in this book will allow you to customize a plan that will strengthen your digestive system and improve your IBS symptoms within the next thirty days. That's a promise.

Chapter 2

Your Digestive System and IBS

If you have IBS, you probably know the location of every public restroom between your home and your place of work. You may avoid social occasions or excuse yourself early from dinner parties to return home and spend hours suffering through abdominal cramping and diarrhea. You may fear mealtime, aware that a forkful of the wrong food can wreak havoc in your digestive system for the rest of the day.

While many people spend a great deal of time learning how to cope with IBS, they often devote little time to learning about IBS and how it affects their digestive system. In this chapter, we will review how the digestive system should work—and what happens when the system breaks down and a person develops IBS.

HOW YOUR DIGESTIVE SYSTEM WORKS

Your digestive system is much more than just your stomach and intestines. It's a complex system of organs that secrete enzymes, contract muscles, and convert the food you eat into the energy your body needs. Ideally, the transit time—the length of time food remains in your body from the moment you eat it to the moment it is excreted as waste—should be twelve to eighteen hours. Problems arise when food moves too quickly or too slowly through the digestive system.

Into the Mouth

The digestive process begins before you take your first bite of food. The sight, smell, and thought of food stimulates the flow of saliva in your mouth. The lining of your mouth contains three pairs of large salivary glands, which together produce about three pints of saliva daily. Each set of glands has a different purpose:

- **The parotid glands** are located in your cheeks, just under your earlobes. Pressure from your molars or the taste of salty or bitter foods causes these glands to excrete a potent saliva that contains the enzyme amylase. Amylase begins to convert starches into sugars that your body can use. As you chew, you can actually taste the food getting sweeter. Saliva from the parotid glands also contains antibodies that protect the body from infection.

- **The submandibular glands** lie in the back of your mouth, along each side of your lower jawbone and deep beneath your tongue. These glands are activated by sour or fatty foods. They produce a thick saliva to help you swallow.

- **The sublingual glands** are located in tissue at the floor of your mouth, just below your tongue. They produce a thin saliva that helps dilute sugar. Sublingual glands are triggered by sweet foods and the natural sugars in fruits and vegetables.

Once you take a bite of food, your salivary glands kick into high gear, pumping out juices that begin to chemically break down the food. Not all the work is chemical, though. Your teeth crunch and grind the food, while your tongue mixes it with the saliva. This chewing and churning transforms a bite of food into what's called a bolus—a soft, moist, rounded mixture suitable for swallowing.

Down the Esophagus

You control what you put into your mouth, how long you chew it, and when you swallow, but after you swallow, your central nervous system takes over the digestive process. When you swallow, muscles in your mouth and throat propel food through a relaxed ring of muscle (the upper esophageal sphincter) and down the esophagus, a tube approximately nine inches long, which empties into the stomach. A series of synchronized contractions forces the food toward the stomach. This process of moving food using waves of muscle contractions is called peristalsis, a process that continues throughout the digestive system.

When food reaches the lower end of your esophagus, the lower esophageal sphincter opens, allowing the food to pass into the stomach. When you're not eating, this muscle valve remains tightly sealed to keep stomach acid from flowing backward (regurgitating) into your esophagus and causing heartburn.

Enter the Stomach

The stomach is a hollow, muscular pouch that lies in the upper left corner of your abdomen, just under your ribs. The stomach measures approximately six to eight inches in length by three to four inches in width; it can expand to hold about one gallon of food and liquid. When the stomach is empty, its tissues fold in on themselves, similar to a collapsed accordion.

In the stomach, food is churned and broken into smaller particles before it is gradually released into the small intestine. Your stomach readies itself for digestion before the first bite of food arrives. At the sight and smell of food, your brain sends messages to the stomach, triggering the release of acetylcholine, a chemical that starts stomach contractions and signals the gastric glands to produce digestive juices. Under normal conditions, your stomach produces two to three quarts of gastric juices every day.

When food enters from the esophagus, muscles in the upper stomach relax to let it in. The stomach walls, which are lined with three layers of powerful muscles, then begin churning the food, mixing it into smaller and smaller pieces. Gastric juices pour out of tiny openings connected to glands that line your stomach. These enzymes help break down food into a thick, creamy fluid called chyme.

Hydrochloric acid is one of many gastric juices. This helpful but corrosive acid could dissolve your stomach itself if it weren't for the sticky alkaline mucus clinging to your stomach walls. Hydrochloric acid kills harmful bacteria and microorganisms swallowed with the food.

The presence of hydrochloric acid and pepsin in the stomach is essential to proper digestion. For many people, the bloating, cramping, and diarrhea associated with IBS are caused by low levels of hydrochloric acid in the stomach. The level of stomach hydrochloric acid declines with age. Some people experience a significant decline as early as the twenties; more than 30 percent of all people over age sixty have inadequate levels of hydrochloric acid in their stomachs.

Once the food is well mixed, muscle contractions push the chyme down toward the pyloric valve, which leads to the upper portion of the small intestine known as the duodenum. The pyloric valve opens just enough to allow about an eighth of an ounce of food at a time into the duodenum.

On to the Small Intestine (With a Little Help from the Pancreas, Liver, and Gallbladder)

The small intestine is your body's main digestive organ, a twenty-two-foot-long twisting tube that fills much of your abdomen. In the small intestine, the chemical breakdown of food is completed and most nutrients are absorbed into the bloodstream. The first part of the small intestine, the twelve-inch-long duodenum, receives digestive juices from three organs: the pancreas, liver, and gallbladder.

- **Pancreas:** The pancreas is a soft, pink gland that lies in the upper abdomen, behind the lower part of your stomach. The pancreas produces the hormones insulin and glucagons, which help regulate metabolism and blood sugar levels; it also produces digestive enzymes that break down proteins, carbohydrates, and fats.

- **Liver:** Located on the right side of the body beneath the rib cage, the liver is a virtual chemical factory that performs more than five hundred functions. This organ—which is nearly the size of a football—stores nutrients, produces cholesterol, and filters out the toxic chemicals found in the foods we eat. The liver also produces bile, a watery, yellowish green solution that assists with the digestion of fats.

- **Gallbladder:** The gallbladder is a small, transparent sac adjacent to the liver that stores and concentrates bile. The gallbladder is about three inches long and holds about two ounces of bile. The liver continuously produces about two pints of bile each day; when your body isn't digesting food, the excess bile drains into bile ducts and backs up into the gallbladder. In the gallbladder, the water found in the bile is absorbed, turning the stored bile into a concentrated, potent solution. When fatty foods enter the duodenum, a hormone signals the gallbladder to contract and release the stored bile into the duodenum.

Flushed with digestive juices from the pancreas, liver, and gallbladder, as well as other juices secreted in the walls of the small intestine itself, digestion quickly reaches a peak. The chemical reactions change proteins into amino acids, fats into glycerin and fatty acids, and starches and sugars into glucose.

Once it is broken down into components that your body can absorb, the food moves into the second portion of the small intestine, the jejunum, which is about eight feet long. Finally, it moves to the third and final portion of the small intestine, the ileum, which is about twelve feet long. In the jejunum and ileum, the body absorbs nutrients through the cell walls. The journey of food through the small intestine generally takes between thirty minutes and three hours, depending on the composition of the meal.

Finally, the Colon and Anus

The colon, also known as the large intestine, stores and removes waste that your body can't digest. The colon is about six feet long; it almost completely frames the perimeter of the small intestine. When food enters the colon, it passes through the ileocecal valve, which opens only one way, so that food waste in the colon can't flow back into the small intestine.

Approximately two quarts of liquid waste enter the colon from the small intestine each day. By the time food residue reaches the colon, the body has absorbed nearly all the nutrients it can. What remain are water, electrolytes, and waste products, such as plant fiber, bacteria, and dead cells shed from the lining of your digestive tract.

During the twelve hours or so that food waste passes through the colon, your body absorbs nearly all the water from the waste. Although it is replete with bacteria, the waste remains harmless to the body as long as the colon walls are intact. The bacteria can, however, cause certain food products to ferment, producing gas. This gas, called flatus, is mainly an odorless mixture of hydrogen, methane, and carbon dioxide. The odors come from certain foods, especially those rich in sulfur, such as garlic and cabbage, and those with sulfur-based preservatives, such as bread, beer, and potato chips.

Muscle contractions force the waste through the colon and separate it into small segments. After a meal, segments of waste are pressed together to form stool, which is then pushed down toward the rectum. When the rectal walls stretch, they signal the brain that it is time to release stool. If you wait to release the stool, your body will continue to absorb water, causing the stool to become hard, compact, and difficult to pass.

The sphincter muscle in your anus is the final valve in the digestive system. When the sphincter muscle relaxes, the rectal walls contract to increase pressure. In some cases, the abdominal muscles are also used to press on the outside of the colon and rectum. When these muscles are contracted, the stool is expelled.

WHEN THE DIGESTIVE SYSTEM BREAKS DOWN: UNDERSTANDING IBS

When the system functions normally, most people give little thought to their digestion. But when the symptoms of IBS appear, many people become preoccupied with how it works.

Though most of my patients with IBS feel as if they are alone in their suffering, IBS affects forty million Americans a year. Women are affected twice as often as men. IBS is responsible for more than three million visits to physicians yearly, and it is one of the leading causes of lost work and school time. Often IBS is just a mild annoyance, but for some people it can be disabling. They may be unable to go to social events, to hold a job, or to travel even short distances. For these people, IBS has a dramatic impact on overall quality of life.

IBS causes a great deal of discomfort and distress, but it does not cause permanent harm to the intestines and does not lead to intestinal bleeding of the bowel or to serious disease, such as cancer. It is characterized by the following symptoms:

- Abdominal cramping
- Gassiness
- Bloating
- Mucus with stool
- Diarrhea (frequent loose stools)

- Constipation (difficult, infrequent bowel movements)
- Alternation between diarrhea and constipation

NOTE: *Symptoms of IBS do not necessarily include bleeding, fever, weight loss, or persistent severe pain; if you experience these symptoms, contact your doctor immediately.*

Could You Have Something More Serious?

The symptoms of IBS resemble many other more serious digestive disorders, such as inflammatory bowel disease. You should consult a doctor to rule out more serious conditions prior to using the information presented in this book. Chapter 14, "When It Isn't IBS," may help you identify some of the subtle distinctions between IBS and other more serious digestive problems.

THE CAUSES OF IBS

IBS is considered a functional disorder because there is no sign of disease when the colon is examined. In other words, the digestive tract looks normal, but it does not function normally.

At one time, doctors attributed IBS to stress alone, but studies suggest both a functional (physiological) and an emotional (psychological) basis for IBS. Researchers have found that ordinary events such as eating and distension from gas will cause the colon muscles of a person with IBS to spasm much more easily than in someone who does not have IBS.

Certain foods trigger IBS symptoms in susceptible people.

Food sensitivities and food allergies (discussed in detail in chapter 4) play a very important role. Hypersensitivity to dairy products is one of the most common IBS triggers. Repeated exposure to these irritating foods can cause a cascade of gastrointestinal problems, ultimately weakening the digestive system and leaving a person vulnerable to chronic IBS.

THE ACID–ALKALINE BALANCE

An imbalance in body chemistry can also exacerbate the symptoms of IBS. Specifically, the tissues in the body can become too acidic, leading to irritation and inflammation. The body's acid–alkaline level is measured on a 14-point pH scale, with 7.0 being neutral. Numbers below 7.0 are acidic, while those above 7.0 are alkaline (or basic). Scientifically, the pH represents the number of positively charged hydrogen ions in a substance. When it comes to IBS, knowing the pH level of your blood and urine can provide a good idea of your digestive health.

The body does not have a single ideal pH level. Different areas of the body have different target pH levels. For example, the blood and tissues should be slightly alkaline, the urine should be neutral or slightly acidic, and the stomach should be somewhat acidic. (The pH of saliva is highly variable.) The body strives to maintain a steady pH level, especially in the blood, similar to the way the body strives to maintain a temperature near the 98.6-degree Fahrenheit mark. When you are healthy, your blood pH is 7.365, or very slightly alkaline.

When the body is too acidic, every cell in the body is affected. In the digestive system, acidity changes can contribute to IBS, causing a cascade of changes including yeast overgrowth, high levels of imbalanced intestinal bacteria, and food allergies. When combating high levels of acid in foods, the blood draws alkaline minerals (such as sodium, potassium, calcium, and magnesium) from the tissues in order to neutralize the acid; in this way, an acidic diet can lead to nutrient deficiencies.

Excess acid also compromises the digestive tract to the point that the naturally occurring yeast, *Candida albicans,* grows in excess, causing the symptoms of IBS as well as other chronic health complaints. In fact, yeast overgrowth has been blamed for dry skin, mood swings, rheumatoid arthritis, low blood sugar, and dozens of other health problems. (Yeast overgrowth is discussed in detail in chapter 6.)

The body's pH can be properly balanced by eating an alkaline diet (described in chapter 7) and by taking certain supplements (described in chapter 11). Taking these healthful steps will not only improve your overall health, but also relieve your IBS symptoms.

You can actually measure the improvement in your systemic pH levels at home by using paper pH test strips, available at most pharmacies. The strips change color when dipped in a urine sample, and the strips are then matched to a color chart to determine the pH of the urine. (Test the urine first thing in the morning to get an accurate reading.) You can retest every few days as you implement the advice in this book, and you will see your pH improve—in addition to feeling a dramatic improvement in your IBS symptoms.

DIAGNOSING IBS

Most doctors misapply the diagnosis of IBS as a catchall for gastrointestinal complaints without a distinct cause. This approach is wrong. Something is triggering the digestive system's response, and a doctor should work with the patient to determine the cause of the problem. Once the source of the problem is identified, the patient will know what to do to resolve the IBS.

The IBS label is usually applied after a doctor performs several tests to exclude the presence of disease. In most cases, a doctor will take a complete medical history and prescribe a series of laboratory tests. (Chapter 3 includes a complete description of diagnostic tests.) If the doctor rules out a structural or biochemical problem, then a patient is diagnosed as having IBS if the symptoms of IBS (listed above) have occurred for at least twelve weeks (not necessarily consecutive) during the previous year.

YOU DON'T NEED TO TURN TO MEDICATION

If you are able to determine which foods and lifestyle issues are triggering your IBS, you will not have to rely on medications—all of which have side effects—to manage your condition. Medications will do nothing more than mask your symptoms; you need to identify and eliminate the cause of your bowel discomfort.

That being said, you should be aware of the medications out there that *other* doctors may recommend or prescribe.

Over-the-Counter Medications

Drugstore shelves are crowded with products to control diarrhea, soft stools, and gas. While many products may temporarily relieve your symptoms, they will do nothing to help your body regain the balance required for improved digestive health.

• **Antidiarrheals:** Loperamide (Imodium) slows the rate at which food leaves your intestines, and increases intestinal water and iron (sodium) absorption to help solidify stool. Other antidiarrheals, such as bismuth (Pepto-Bismol), also may relieve diarrhea and the urgency to have a bowel movement. You need to be careful not to use antidiarrheal medications too often or too long. Overuse can lead to or worsen constipation.

• **Fiber supplements:** Natural fiber supplements (such as Metamucil or Citrucel) tend to relieve constipation in one to three days. They must be taken with plenty of water so that they do not become constipating. In addition, many patients have sensitivity to psyllium (a common ingredient in fiber supplements), so it can cause inflammation.

• **Laxatives:** Laxatives include stool softeners (such as Colace and Surfak), saline laxatives (such as Phillips' Milk of Magnesia, which increases water content in the stool), and stimulant laxatives (such as Dulcolax, Ex-Lax, and Senokot). Regular use of laxatives can aggravate constipation because you can become dependent on laxatives for bowel movements.

Prescription Medications

Doctors routinely prescribe medications for IBS. Commonly prescribed medications include:

• **Zelnorm,** a new drug that has been advertised on TV recently, is a 5-HT^4 receptor agonist for IBS and recurrent abdominal pain. It is claimed that this medicine works on the source of the problem, but no one has a Zelnorm deficiency.

• **Alosetron:** This is the first medication approved by the Food and Drug Administration specifically for the treatment of IBS. Alosetron (Lotronex) is a nerve receptor antagonist that relaxes the colon and slows the movement of waste through the colon. It's especially useful if you have diarrhea or alternating diarrhea and constipation, rather than just constipation. The medication also helps relieve abdominal pain and cramping. Constipation is a reported side effect.

• **Smooth-muscle relaxants:** Anticholinergic (antispasmodic) drugs such as hyoscyamine sulfate (Levsin) and dicyclomine (Bentyl) may help relax intestinal muscles and relieve muscle spasms. However, the data supporting their use for IBS are limited. These drugs are not approved by the FDA for use in the treatment of IBS, but many doctors prescribe them for the condition nonetheless. The medications have common reported side effects including urinary retention, accelerated heart rate, blurred vision, and dry mouth.

• **Antidepressants:** In addition to relieving depression, these drugs can help relieve abdominal pain and diarrhea or constipation. Your doctor may recommend a tricyclic antidepressant or a selective serotonin reuptake inhibitor (SSRI). The tricyclic agents amitriptyline (Elavil), imipramine (Tofranil), and doxepin (Sinequan) are most frequently prescribed for IBS patients with diarrhea. Tricyclic antidepressants may cause drowsiness, dry mouth, and constipation. The SSRIs fluoxetine (Prozac) and paroxetine (Paxil) are most frequently prescribed for pain with constipation in IBS patients. SSRIs can cause nausea, cramping, and diarrhea.

I do not recommend the use of these medications in the treatment of IBS. To heal your body and develop gastrointestinal balance, you must stop irritating your system and allow it to heal. The information in this book will help you identify what foods trigger your IBS, so that you can avoid them. In my extensive experience treating patients with IBS, I have found that most people are sensitive to one or more foods; when these foods are eliminated from their diet, their symptoms improve. The cure for IBS is prevention: Avoid the foods that cause the problem and your body will heal itself.

Chapter 3

Do You Have IBS?

IBS isn't a subtle disorder. The chronic episodes of bloating, gas, abdominal cramping, diarrhea, constipation, or alternating bouts of both diarrhea and constipation provide all the evidence most people need to know that they have IBS.

As mentioned earlier, however, symptoms of IBS can resemble those of other more serious conditions. To confirm the diagnosis of IBS and to rule out other illnesses, a doctor should perform a series of tests on your gastrointestinal system. This chapter describes the tests I recommend to my patients, as well as the tests often used by traditional doctors. I do support the use of conventional diagnostic tests, but I rarely use them because most of the patients who come to see me have already visited one or more doctors and undergone a full battery of diagnostic tests.

A DIFFERENT APPROACH TO DIAGNOSIS

A patient came from Canada to see me after he had been diagnosed with colitis; his colon was so badly ulcerated that the doctor recommended that a portion of it be surgically removed. The man had been on cortisone therapy for eighteen months, but he had not found any significant permanent relief of his symptoms. His doctors had not made any dietary recommendations. The first time he came to my office, I performed a simple blood test and discovered that the man was hypersensitive to the pesticides on the fruits he was eating, which was one of the major triggers of his colitis. He was also sensitive to many other foods and chemicals. I changed his diet and put him on oral and intravenous vitamin therapy. In four weeks, his colitis had improved greatly and he no longer needed surgery.

This patient's experience is not uncommon. Many of my patients follow their doctor's advice to the letter, but fail to improve because the recommendations are not customized to meet that individual's needs. When a patient comes to see me, I first find out if all the conventional diagnostic tests for gastrointestinal disease have been done (these standard tests are described later in this chapter). If other illnesses have been ruled out, I typically conduct three types of tests: a gastric analysis, a biological terrain assessment, and antibody tests for food and chemical hypersensitivities.

Gastric Analysis Test

I recommend that all my patients with IBS receive a gastric analysis test, also known as the Heidelberg test, to measure the pH levels in the stomach and small intestine. Many cases of IBS begin with pH imbalances in the stomach. If the pH of the gastric juices in the stomach rises above 3.0, then the stomach does not have enough acid, creating an environment that allows the overgrowth of yeast and parasites and a bacteria, known as *Helicobacter pylori,* which contributes to the formation of ulcers. Many antacids and prescription medications used to treat IBS increase the gastric pH to excessively high levels, setting the stage for the development of secondary digestive problems.

To perform this noninvasive test, a patient comes to the office after a twelve-hour fast. The patient swallows a small capsule with a device to measure pH and a tiny high-frequency transmitter in it. The patient wears a belt, which is wired with an antenna system that accepts signals from the transmitter and feeds the data into a pH gastrogram machine. The transmitter also provides information on emptying time, to see if the stomach is emptying too fast or too slow. (Food left in the stomach too long will ferment; food that leaves the stomach too quickly can contain undissolved proteins, which are large undigested molecules that can trigger immune and autoimmune responses. Undigested proteins would not cause problems if they were broken down properly into amino acids in the stomach during normal digestion.)

Some doctors attempt to get similar information on stomach pH by inserting a tube down the patient's throat to obtain a sample of gastric juice; the Heidelberg machine is obviously much less invasive. The procedure usually takes from forty-five minutes to an hour.

Biological Terrain Assessment: Blood, Saliva, Urine Test

Because IBS can be caused by an imbalance in the body's pH, I recommend that all my patients with IBS undergo a biological terrain assessment (BTA), a test that examines the biochemistry of the blood, saliva, and urine. If the body's pH falls out of balance, it can create an environment where bacteria, fungi, and viruses can flourish. (The acid–alkaline balance is discussed in greater detail on page 18.)

If a person is not digesting food properly or is eating too many acidic foods, the body will fall out of balance as the acid builds up in the tissues. A simple urine test can determine if the body is too acidic, because the excess acid will be eliminated in the urine.

Before receiving a BTA test, a patient should fast for twelve hours and collect a specimen of the first morning urine (after 4 A.M.). Patients should not wear lipstick, makeup, lotion, or anything else around the mouth, which could alter the pH of the saliva. For the same reason, the patient should avoid toothbrushing, licking stamps, smoking, or taking any medications during the fasting period.

The test measures the following:

- **Blood pH:** The pH of the blood should remain right around 7.4, or nearly neutral. The body strives to maintain this balance. The body has compensatory mechanisms to keep the pH at a steady level, but these systems can be overstressed when a person consumes a highly acidic diet—which is the typical American diet—on an ongoing basis. A healthy person has enough alkaline in the body to buffer an occasional bout of excess acid, but those who consume high levels of acid at every meal exceed the body's ability to neutralize it. When this happens, the body depletes its reserves of potassium and magnesium, but it cannot neutralize the acid as fast as it is accumulating. This acid imbalance leads to vitamin, mineral, and nutrient deficits, which contribute to IBS.

- **Urine pH:** In a healthy person, the urine pH is 6.5. If the pH falls below this level, the urine is too acidic.
- **Saliva pH:** The pH of saliva should be less than 7.0. When the digestive system falls out of balance, some of the enzymes present in saliva break down, undermining the first phase of digestion, which begins with the saliva.

In addition, the BTA test can provide information on antioxidant levels, demineralization, and other biochemical markers of overall health.

Antibody Tests for Food Allergies and Hypersensitivities

Food and chemical hypersensitivities are a major cause of IBS symptoms. Food and chemical sensitivities are discussed in detail in chapter 4; in order to determine whether food and chemicals play a role in a patient's IBS, I encourage most patients to undergo blood tests for food and chemical sensitivities. This test is a sample of blood drawn and examined for antibodies indicating an immune response to foods and chemicals. The most common culprits include dairy products and gluten.

This blood test, known as a RAST test (radioallergosorbent test), can be used to identify both food and environmental allergens. In my practice I use both the RAST-IgE (which detects immediate allergens) and the RAST-IgG (which detects delayed allergens). The IgE test is an excellent test for environmental allergens, but it is a less accurate tool for identifying food allergens unless they are IgE mediated. While some doctors challenge the validity of the RAST-IgG test (largely due to reliability problems with a less sensitive test known as the modified RAST, which was widely used in the past), I believe it provides additional information to help patients identify the trigger foods causing their IBS. These tests also can eliminate some of the time required to conduct elimination and rotation diets to identify food allergens by monitoring the diet alone.

It is possible to determine food allergens by restricting most foods from the diet, then adding them back one by one while watching for symptoms, but this can be a painfully difficult process. In addition, this elimination diet approach can be very unreliable, since many foods contain more than one ingredient, so the patient will not know exactly what food triggered the response. I have also had patients who thought they were allergic to a certain type of fruit or vegetable, only to learn from the blood test that they did not respond to the produce itself but rather to a pesticide residue left on the produce. A patient could not learn this without turning to a blood test. Similarly, many patients are allergic to molds that grow on wheat rather than the wheat itself.

Another test known as the ELISA/ACT (enzyme-linked immunosorbent assay) test can be very useful to patients with IBS. The ELISA/ACT test identifies hypersensitive food reactions to chemicals and preservatives. I tend to turn to the ELISA test if a patient with IBS continues to have symptoms after we have eliminated the major food triggers detected by basic testing. In my experience, patients are apt to be allergic to common foods like wheat and common preservatives in our food, such as benzoic acid.

For most patients, most or all of the costs of these tests are covered by health insurance. (The cost depends on how many allergens we test for; the price typically ranges from $300 to

$1,000 or so.) ELISA/ACT Testing can be reached at 800-553-5472.

Comprehensive Stool Test

The final test I recommend, if needed, for my patients with IBS is a comprehensive stool test, which looks for parasites, yeast cultures, and inappropriate bacteria, all of which can contribute to the development of IBS symptoms. Other stool tests may look for white blood count and red blood count, as well as inflammatory markers. While some conventional doctors perform stool tests, they tend to look for a narrow range of parasites.

If you want your doctor to prescribe a comprehensive stool test, I recommend the use of Great Smokies Diagnostic Laboratory (800-522-4762) or Diagnos-Techs (800-87-TESTS). These labs offer a far more thorough exam than most facilities.

TESTS MOST DOCTORS PERFORM

When a patient complains of IBS, a doctor must conduct some diagnostic tests to eliminate the possibility of other serious illnesses that have the same symptoms as IBS. In some cases, a doctor may be able to rule out most conditions after conducting a complete physical exam and taking a medical history. While the specific tests your doctor recommends will depend on your health profile, the following is a rundown of common diagnostic tests.

Blood Tests

Almost all patients receive blood tests as a first step in diagnosing a digestive disorder because they are simple to do and they provide a general idea of what's going on inside your body. You may receive several tests, including the following:

- **Complete blood count (CBC):** This test measures a number of blood properties, including the number of red and white cells. A reduction in red blood cells (anemia) may be associated with gastrointestinal bleeding; an elevation in white blood cells may indicate an infection or inflammation, including infection and inflammation of the digestive tract.

- **Blood chemistry:** This test measures the electrolyte levels in the blood. Chronic diarrhea or vomiting can cause an abnormality in the levels of the electrolytes sodium and potassium in the blood. A severely low level of potassium can put you at risk of heart problems. In addition, blood chemistry tests can examine blood sugar levels and markers of kidney and liver function.

Urine Tests

Most doctors ask for a urine sample, which is then screened for abnormal levels of protein (a sign of kidney problems), glucose (a sign of diabetes), and blood (a sign of infection or inflammation). Some doctors also test the pH level of the urine and look for ketones in the urine, which are a by-product of fat metabolism and can be present in people with diabetes. Urinalysis is another routine gateway test that can provide important information about a patient's overall health.

Stool Tests

Most doctors do not conduct stool tests on their patients with IBS, and those who do typically conduct incomplete analysis. A comprehensive stool analysis should include:

- **Parasite test:** A doctor should request a stool sample to check for parasites or bacteria (or for traces of their associated toxins), especially if your IBS symptoms include severe diarrhea.

- **Hemoccult test:** Another common stool test is a fecal occult blood test (hemoccult test). This test looks for hidden (occult) blood that may be linked to cancer or other diseases that can cause intestinal bleeding, such as ulcers or inflammatory bowel disease. A fecal occult blood test may be a routine part of colorectal cancer screening for people over age fifty. Not all cancers bleed, however, and those that do often bleed intermittently. It is possible to have a negative test result even though cancer is present. Certain foods also contain chemicals that can produce a false reading; broccoli, cauliflower, and undercooked red meat can cause a false reading, indicating blood in stool when there isn't any. Vitamin C supplements can mask a positive reaction, keeping the strip from turning color when blood is present.

Radiological Procedures

Conventional doctors routinely prescribe X-rays to detect diseases that can cause symptoms similar to those of IBS. The type of X-ray you receive will depend on the location of your symptoms:

• **Upper gastrointestinal X-ray:** This test employs a series of X-ray images to look for abnormalities in the esophagus, stomach, and the first part of the small intestine (duodenum). After an evening of fasting to clear food from the digestive system, the patient swallows a thick, white liquid containing barium, an alkaline chemical that temporarily coats the lining of the digestive tract to make it show up more clearly on X-ray films. You also may be asked to swallow a gas-producing substance (such as sodium bicarbonate), which will inflate the stomach, separating its folds and offering a better view of the inner lining.

The radiologist watches on a video monitor as the barium moves through the stomach, revealing any malfunctions or abnormalities in the digestive system. For example, this procedure can show if the muscles that control swallowing are functioning properly, and it can reveal tumors, ulcers, or a narrowing (stricture) of the esophagus, all of which can cause digestive symptoms.

The entire procedure may take one to two hours. The barium passes out with the stool, creating whitish stools for several days. Constipation is a common side effect of the procedure; drink plenty of fluids for a few days afterward. This is a routine screening test for patients with IBS symptoms.

• **Small-intestine (small-bowel) X-ray:** If your doctor wants a more complete set of X-rays, he or she may expand the upper gastrointestinal (GI) X-ray to include the entire small intestine. This procedure may take up to four hours. This test is used in much the same way as the traditional upper GI X-ray.

• **Colon X-ray:** Also known as a barium enema, the colon X-ray allows a doctor to x-ray the entire colon to detect ulcers, narrowed areas, growths along the lining of the colon (polyps), small pouches in the lining (diverticula), cancer, and other abnormalities that could cause digestive problems.

For one to two days before the test, the patient must consume only clear liquids, such as broth, gelatin, coffee, tea, and other beverages, in order to empty the colon. Laxatives or enemas are then used to clear out the remainder of the colon. On the day of the exam, barium is placed in the colon through a tube inserted in the rectum. The barium coats the lining of the colon so that the images will appear on an X-ray. In some cases, the radiologist will inject air into the colon to improve the image. The exam typically lasts about twenty minutes. It is routinely administered to IBS patients to rule out more serious problems.

- **Computed tomography or CT scan:** Computed tomography combines X-rays with computer technology to produce a clear, three-dimensional picture of your internal organs, bone, and other tissues. It is an effective way to diagnose tumors, blood- or fluid-filled cysts, or infections (abscesses) inside the body. During the procedure, the patient lies on a platform that slides into an X-ray scanner. The scanner takes a series of very thin X-rays from many angles while it rotates around the body. Using these images, the computer creates a three-dimensional picture that can be dissected layer by layer. A CT scan of the abdomen and pelvis can identify abnormalities in the pancreas, liver, kidneys, intestines, gallbladder, and bile ducts.

Prior to the procedure, the patient must fast overnight, then drink or receive an injection of an iodine-based liquid that makes the organs show up more clearly on the X-ray. This test can reveal structural problems that could cause symptoms similar to those of IBS. Most patients receive an X-ray series, followed by a CT scan if a problem is suspected or identified in one of the procedures.

Ultrasound

This test is not usually used on patients who complain of IBS, unless there is reason to suspect problems with the organs as well. Typically, ultrasound is used to examine the liver, pancreas, gallbladder, kidneys, and other abdominal organs. It is often used to detect gallstones or to reveal the shape, texture, and makeup of tumors and cysts.

Ultrasound procedures combine high-frequency sound waves and computer technology to produce pictures of the internal organs. During the procedure, the patient lies on an examining table while a technician places a wandlike device (transducer) on the abdomen. The transducer sends and receives inaudible sound waves that reflect off the tissues in the body, much the same way that sonar reflects off the bottom of the ocean. A computer converts the sound waves into a moving, two-dimensional image. The exam is painless and usually takes about thirty minutes.

Endoscopy

It is possible to look inside the digestive tract by using an endoscope, a thin, flexible tube with a fiber-optic light and a tiny electronic camera. To explore the digestive tract, the scope can be slipped down through the mouth, esophagus, stomach, and upper small intestine, or it can be inserted up through the anus, rectum, and colon. When used to examine the lower gastrointestinal tract, an endoscope is referred to as a colonoscope or sigmoidoscope; a sigmoidoscope is shorter than a colonoscope.

• **Upper endoscopy:** This procedure (esophagogastroduodenoscopy, or EGD) allows a doctor to look inside the esophagus, stomach, and duodenum to identify inflamed tissue, ulcers, or abnormal growths. Small instruments also may be inserted through the tube to remove noncancerous growths (polyps) or to take tissue samples (biopsies). The patient must fast for four to six hours before the test. An anesthetic spray is used to numb the throat and prevent gagging; in many cases, mild sedation is also used.

This test can reveal abnormalities that won't show up as well on an X-ray image, such as inflamed or damaged esophageal tissue from reflux or stomach acid (gastritis, which is frequently seen with IBS), and small ulcers or tumors in the stomach or duodenum. The procedure takes about thirty minutes, but it may take an hour or more to recover from the sedatives. This test is often used for IBS patients to rule out ulcers or serious inflammatory conditions in the digestive tract.

• **Colonoscopy:** This procedure allows a doctor to inspect the colon for abnormalities, such as bleeding, inflammation, tumors, pouches, or narrowed areas; it also allows the doctor to take biopsy samples, remove polyps, treat bleeding sites, and stretch narrowed areas. The colon must be empty for the exam, so the patient switches to a liquid-only diet for two days and uses either laxatives or enemas to clear the colon.

Prior to the exam, the patient receives a sedative and pain reliever. The patient lies on the left side, and the colonoscope is inserted into the rectum and moved through the colon. The device has a tube that allows the doctor to inflate the colon for a better view. The procedure usually takes between fifteen and sixty minutes.

A so-called virtual colonoscopy or computed tomographic colography provides two- and three-dimensional pictures of the colon and rectum without using a colonoscope. The procedure also requires that the colon be clear of stool. During the procedure, the colon is inflated using a small catheter and a CT scanner. The procedure typically takes less than ten minutes and can identify polyps that are larger than half an inch. If suspicious areas are located, traditional colonoscopy is used to follow up, provide biopsies, and remove polyps. Colonoscopy is a routine test for people with IBS symptoms, and can be very effective at identifying problems in the lower digestive system. It is the classic test used to diagnose colitis.

- **Sigmoidoscopy:** This procedure is similar to a colonoscopy, except that it involves only the rectum and last portion of the colon (the sigmoid colon), rather than the entire colon. Typically, sigmoidoscopy does not require sedation, and it takes only about ten minutes.

Sigmoidoscopy is used more often than colonoscopy as a diagnostic test for people with IBS. It is a routine cancer screening test for people over age fifty. In some cases, sigmoidoscopy is combined with a full colon X-ray, which shows the entire colon. If polyps are detected during the exam, most doctors recommend a colonoscopy to remove the polyps and examine the entire colon for additional polyps. I recommend the use of colonoscopy rather than sigmoidoscopy when doing a lower GI test because it examines more surface area, it is more extensive, and polyps can be removed at the time of the procedure.

Transit Studies

If a patient has ongoing abdominal pain, nausea, vomiting, constipation, or diarrhea and other diagnostic tests have not revealed a cause, many doctors will order transit studies to measure how fast food passes through the digestive system. If digestive muscles or nerves aren't working properly, food may move through the system too quickly or too slowly. These tests are less common than those described above; they may confirm that a patient has a slow transit time, but they do not suggest a cause for the problem.

- **Gastric emptying:** This test evaluates how quickly the stomach empties food into the small intestine. It is typically used if a patient experiences unexplained vomiting or complains of feeling full after eating a moderate amount of food. After fasting overnight, a patient visits the doctor and eats bread, a glass of milk, and eggs containing a few drops of a slightly radioactive tracer substance. Gamma-radiation cameras then photograph the eggs as they pass through the stomach; the images don't show the internal organs, only the radioactive eggs.

If the stomach is emptying normally, 11 to 39 percent of the eggs leave the stomach in one hour, 40 percent to 76 percent at two hours, and 84 percent to 98 percent at four hours.

- **Gastric emptying and small-bowel transit:** This test is the same as the gastric emptying test, except that an additional series of pictures is taken at six hours. If your small intestine is moving the food normally, 46 percent to 98 percent of the eggs will have passed through your small intestine by this time and be in your colon.

• **Whole-gut transit:** During this test, the patient swallows a capsule containing a radioactive tracer element that is designed to remain intact until it reaches the upper colon. The patient eats the same egg breakfast and has the same pictures, with an additional image taken twenty-four hours later. At this time, the capsule should have released its tracer element, which should be seen mixed in with food residue in the middle or lower colon. If the tracer element remains at the beginning of the colon, the colon isn't propelling food waste normally.

• **Colon transit:** This test is often used for people who complain of severe, persistent constipation. The procedure resembles the whole-gut transit study, without the breakfast. A picture is taken at the time the capsule is swallowed, and another one four hours later. At the time of the four-hour picture, the capsule should be in the beginning of the colon. You need to return the next day for a twenty-four-hour picture to visualize how far the tracer element has progressed. As in the whole-gut study, if the element hasn't made it to your middle or lower colon, your colon isn't propelling food fast enough.

While few patients require a full battery of tests, most doctors prescribe enough tests to ensure that the IBS symptoms are not due to a more serious gastrointestinal problem. There is no need to wait for diagnostic tests to be performed to improve your digestive health. I recommend that my patients take the steps described in this book to balance their digestive system and improve their diet immediately, without waiting for definitive test results. In my experience, many IBS patients feel much better by taking a few simple steps—most notably eliminating dairy, gluten, and yeast from the diet—even if they have not fully analyzed their responses to specific foods. More often than not, patients who follow the program feel better than they have in years when they return to my office for a follow-up appointment after a week or two.

FINDING THE RIGHT DOCTOR

While this book contains many suggestions you can try on your own, you need to establish a relationship with a medical professional who can monitor your overall health and provide the necessary diagnostic tests discussed earlier. If possible, it is best to develop a relationship with a doctor before you reach a crisis state, so that the physician will be familiar with you and your medical issues long before you enter the office with a serious concern.

As a medical doctor with expertise in both conventional and alternative medicine, I appreciate the virtues of both approaches to healing. Natural medicine differs from mainstream medicine in its basic approach to healing. Simply put, conventional medicine treats and manages the symptoms of disease (it strives to make you feel better), while natural medicine treats the whole person. Natural medicine puts an emphasis on preventing disease, while conventional medicine has only recently begun to appreciate the link between lifestyle choices and overall health.

Natural medicine is based on the simple but profound premise that the human body is designed to heal itself. The medical professional's role is to help the body heal itself; in the case of IBS, this means learning which foods to avoid, which foods to eat, and which nutrients may be required to ensure that the body has the building blocks it needs to rebuild itself.

This approach to healing IBS works, but it also requires that you, the patient, make a commitment to your own health. Some patients want to take a pill and feel better so that they can go back to their old ways of eating. You must take responsibility for your health by adopting a healthy diet and lifestyle. A balanced digestive system is possible, but most people will have to make some adjustments in the way they eat, exercise, and manage stress in order to achieve this goal.

Many IBS patients describe the relationship with their doctor as frustrating and unsatisfactory. Too many doctors do not view IBS as a legitimate medical condition and dismiss the condition out of hand. This is not acceptable; you deserve to work with a doctor who is respectful, empathic, and well educated about various treatment options. To find out about an individual physician's philosophy of healing, you need to set up an interview and ask a range of questions.

There are several types of physicians to choose from:

- **Gastroenterologists** are medical doctors who specialize in the treatment of disorders of the digestive system. They have knowledge about virtually all treatments for IBS and other gastrointestinal problems, but not all of them are open to alternative treatments and therapies. In my experience, most gastroenterologists will resort to the use of drug therapy in the treatment of IBS.

- **Family practice doctors** are medical doctors who specialize in the treatment of all family members, from infants to geriatric patients. They have general knowledge of treatments for IBS, but they refer their patients with special health problems to specialists. Again, most family practice doctors will rely on drug therapy to treat IBS.

• **Internists** are doctors of internal medicine who manage the overall health of adults; many internists refer patients with serious gastrointestinal problems to a gastroenterologist for specialized care. When treating IBS patients, they typically turn to drug therapy.

• **General practitioners** treat the whole patient rather than specializing in the treatment of one body system or condition. While a general practitioner may be able to help treat mild IBS, most work in conjunction with a specialist for chronic or severe digestive problems. They also rely on the use of medications in most cases.

• **Naturopathic physicians** practice natural medicine using a variety of healing techniques, including nutritional supplementation, herbal medicine, homeopathy, and other techniques. Training to become a naturopath resembles traditional medical school, although naturopathic physicians receive the degree *N.D.* (naturopathic doctor) rather than *M.D.* (medical doctor). Standard premed courses must be taken by students at all of the nation's three recognized naturopathic medical schools, Bastyr University, the National College of Naturopathic Medicine, and the Southwest College of Naturopathic Medicine and Health Sciences. Students take many of the same courses as conventional medical students, as well as courses in nutrition, herbal healing, physical medicine, and counseling. Naturopathic physicians do not use prescription medications.

Questions to Ask a Prospective Doctor

Try to find a doctor with whom you can establish an ongoing, helpful relationship. The following questions can help you get to know more about your doctor's overall philosophy. You may be able to discuss some of these matters with the office manager before your appointment.

- What would you do with a patient with my symptoms?
- What diagnostic tests would you recommend to evaluate my condition?
- Do you use vitamin and nutrient therapy?
- What kind of dietary changes do you recommend for people with IBS?
- Do you typically prescribe drugs for people with my condition? What are the side effects of these medications?
- Do you have training in alternative or complementary medicine?
- Do you do any testing for food allergies or sensitivities?
- Are there any new treatments in development for IBS?
- What IBS support groups exist in our area? Which do you recommend?
- How often do I need to see you for follow-up care?

You may be able to get recommendations of qualified doctors in your area from a local IBS support group. You also may seek referrals from one or more of the organizations listed in the resources section at the back of this book.

As with any health care provider, if you aren't satisfied with the treatment you receive, or if you don't feel comfortable with the patient–practitioner relationship, keep looking for a practitioner who offers a better match. Many people with IBS try several physicians before finding one who satisfies their long-term needs.

Once you find a physician, he or she can help you identify some of the foods that may be contributing to your IBS symptoms. The following chapter will explain how food allergies and sensitivities trigger IBS symptoms and how you can identify the offending foods and eliminate them from your diet.

Chapter 4

Understanding Food Sensitivities and Food Allergies

Allergy sufferers need to know their enemies. Hay fever sufferers need to know when to stay indoors to avoid seasonal pollens, people who are allergic to penicillin need to know which antibiotics their doctors prescribe to avoid a serious reaction, and people plagued by IBS need to know which foods may be triggering their diarrhea, cramping, and other symptoms of digestive distress. Unfortunately, most people with IBS don't have any idea which foods tend to tie their intestines in knots, and they aren't sure how to find out. This chapter will help you identify the food allergies that may be contributing to your IBS.

Food allergies and sensitivities are a primary cause of IBS symptoms. When one of my patients has a food hypersensitivity, the immune system overreacts to a substance that is not normally harmful. In the case of a food sensitivity or intolerance, a person suffers from IBS symptoms because the body's immune system attacks the food or chemical and forms antibodies. For a person suffering from IBS, both allergies and sensitivities can disrupt the digestive system and create gastrointestinal anguish.

Conventional doctors accept the idea of food allergies, but they don't utilize the many useful methods of diagnostic testing and treatment. If you have IBS, your doctor should work with you to determine if you have any food sensitivities or allergies, which in my experience are a common aggravation to the digestive system, and a common source of digestive problems.

UNDERSTANDING THE IMMUNE SYSTEM RESPONSE

When a person with an allergy eats an allergenic food, his or her body identifies the food as foreign molecules (known as antigens), and the immune system responds by releasing B lymphocyte cells, which attack the invaders. The immune system also releases into the blood antibodies (or immunoglobins), which allow the white blood cells in the body to identify and kill the offending cells. Antigens can be microorganisms (viruses, yeast, parasites, and bacteria), environmental allergens (dust, pollen, or pet dander, for example), or ingredients in common foods. In some cases the symptoms are mild, such as sneezing or a runny nose, but at other times they can be life threatening in the form of a reaction known as anaphylaxis.

There are two basic types of allergic reactions, immediate and delayed:

- **Immediate reactions:** People who suffer immediate allergic reactions to certain foods exhibit obvious and often life-threatening symptoms minutes to hours after eating an allergenic food; many are forced to carry adrenaline with them in case of accidental exposure to avoid a potentially deadly emergency. Common triggers include shellfish (such as crabs, lobster, or shrimp), nuts (especially peanuts), and cinnamon. Immediate food allergies have a genetic component, and they last a lifetime. They account for about 10 percent of all allergic reactions associated with food.

- **Delayed reactions:** The remaining 90 percent of food allergies involve delayed reactions. These responses, known as either delayed food allergies or food sensitivities, occur from four to forty-eight hours after eating an allergenic food. Because of the delay between the time a food is consumed and the time symptoms arise, diagnosis of delayed food allergies can be very difficult. In addition to foods, you can have delayed allergies to food additives, food coloring, pesticides, heavy metals, and pollutants. Most foods and tap water contain traces of pesticides and industrial chemicals; these substances should not be overlooked as potential allergens when you assess your food sensitivities.

LEARNING FROM YOUR ANTIBODIES

You can identify food allergies in one of two ways: You can carefully monitor your diet and identify food triggers one at a time, or you can have a doctor perform a blood test that will identify specific markers indicating specific food allergies. While both approaches work, I recommend that my patients have the blood test because they can make the necessary adjustments to their diets without a long trial-and-error period.

The blood test essentially examines the antibodies found in the blood and places them into one of several categories. Antibodies, which are made up primarily of amino acids, can be divided into several major classes:

• **IgM:** This is the first antibody produced by the immune system when the body encounters a new irritant or microorganism. These antibodies diminish a few months after exposure.

• **IgG:** These antibodies indicate the body has encountered an offending irritant or organism for a second or subsequent time. IgG antibodies are associated with delayed food reactions.

• **IgE:** These antibodies are most widely known for their involvement with allergies in general. Elevated IgE in the blood is linked to a history of exposure to an allergen. Immediate allergic reactions—hives, swelling, congestion, and the like—result from IgE activity. These antibodies are associated with immediate reactions to allergenic foods, as well as dust, pollen, and other environmental allergens.

• **IgA:** These antibodies protect the nasal and intestinal lining from microorganisms. A saliva test indicating elevated levels of IgA antibodies can indicate a sensitivity to gluten and other irritants. Food allergies occur more often in people with low levels of secretory IgA.

Identifying the types of antibodies in your blood can provide essential information about your digestive health, and can identify both immediate and delayed food reactions. The results can provide a dietary road map of which foods you should avoid to eliminate symptoms of IBS.

HOW YOU CAN IDENTIFY FOOD ALLERGIES ON YOUR OWN

If you do not have access to a doctor who can conduct blood tests for food allergies, you can do some detective work on your own to determine which foods may disrupt your digestive system. No single food allergen triggers IBS in all people, so it's up to you to work through an elimination diet to identify an allergy if you have one. (Almost all the IBS patients in my practice have at least one food allergy.) The task can be difficult, because many people are allergic to more than one food.

There are two ways of conducting an elimination diet. You can either eliminate the single food suspected of causing problems and wait several days to see if your symptoms subside, or you can attempt to systematically test all the foods in your diet. To conduct a full-diet test, you should allow your body to rest for four to seven days; during this period eat only the following foods:

- Fruits (except citrus)
- All vegetables (except corn and tomatoes)
- Brown rice
- Turkey
- Almonds, walnuts, or sunflower seeds

During this "rest" period, your IBS symptoms should greatly subside. Next you will introduce a test food, watching carefully for an increase in IBS symptoms. If you notice an increase in IBS symptoms within two to forty-eight hours, omit this food from your diet for a week, then try introducing it again. If symptoms return again, cut this food from your diet. Introduce a new food every second day. The process is time consuming because it can take a long period of time to identify the offending foods. There is no simple solution, but if you work at it, you may be able to find considerable relief by changing your diet.

During the elimination diet, it is essential to maintain a food diary. Keep records of the date, meal, time, food consumed, and any physical reaction you might have. These records will help you detect patterns in your responses to certain foods. For example, you may find that you experience diarrhea an hour after eating corn or foods containing cornmeal and other corn derivatives.

Some of the most common allergenic foods are dairy products, wheat, oats, eggs, corn, peanuts, shellfish, tomatoes, and strawberries. Common allergenic food additives include FD&C Yellow No. 5, vanillin, sulfites, benzaldehyde, monosodium glutamate, BHT/BHA, and benzoates. If you are allergic to ragweed, you are probably allergic to cantaloupe, which contains some of the same proteins as ragweed. You may want to start your search with these foods.

Symptoms of Delayed Food Allergies

Immediate food allergies give prompt and dramatic evidence of their presence. Delayed food allergies, on the other hand, can be much more subtle and difficult to recognize. By keeping a detailed food journal and recording the foods you eat and how you feel throughout the day, you will be able to recognize the symptoms of a delayed food allergy. (You will find a thirty-day food journal in chapter 12.) The following symptoms can help you determine if you may have an unidentified delayed food allergy:

- Chronic digestive problems, including the symptoms of IBS
- Recurring infections, such as sinusitis, tonsillitis, ear, respiratory, urinary, and so forth
- Recurring inflammatory conditions, such as gastrointestinal inflammation, arthritis, et cetera
- Difficulty losing excess weight
- Unexplained bouts of severe fatigue after eating
- Tendency to hold water that is not associated with the menstrual cycle
- Dark circles under your eyes (sometimes called allergic shiners)
- A horizontal crease under the lower eyelid (as if your skin had been pinched); the crease gets deeper after meals
- Frequent stuffy nose or postnasal drip that lasts for several hours after meals; also clearing your throat frequently after eating
- Chronically swollen glands
- Anxiety and heart palpitations within several hours of eating
- Unexplained skin rashes
- History of gallbladder disease
- History of acne
- History of antibiotic use
- Mental fogginess after eating
- Bouts of low blood sugar
- Headaches

A Quick Self-Test

You can get a general idea if you have a food allergy by testing your pulse after eating a potentially allergenic food. Using a watch with a second hand, take your pulse at the wrist by counting the number of heartbeats for thirty seconds, then double the result. (Your pulse will probably be between fifty-two and seventy beats a minute.) Eat the food you suspect may be a trigger food, and take your pulse again fifteen minutes later. If your pulse is twenty or more beats per minute higher, you probably have an allergy to the food.

Try to test the food in its simplest form. For example, when testing for an allergy to oats, you would want to test plain oat cereal (available at health food stores) rather than commercially prepared oatmeal, which has many other ingredients. This is not a foolproof test, but it does offer an easy way to identify certain problem foods.

FOOD ALLERGIES AND LEAKY GUT SYNDROME

Some delayed food allergies may not be triggered by antibodies at all. Instead, they may be caused by leaky gut syndrome, also known as excessive intestinal permeability. Leaky gut syndrome can result from a number of factors including an overgrowth of yeast or bacteria, infection of the gastrointestinal tract, viral infection, poor nutrition or absorption of nutrients, and genetic predisposition. Bacterial overgrowth can be caused by poor diet and the use of antibiotics.

Of course, the intestinal tract is designed to allow nutrients to pass through it. Problems arise when the digestive system is stressed to the point that the lining of the intestines thins and develops tiny holes, similar to cheesecloth. The condition earned the name *leaky gut* because particles of undigested proteins and other food particles slip through the gastrointestinal lining, where they enter the bloodstream. The immune system identifies these wayward food particles as foreign invaders and initiates a full-blown immune response. This response is believed to create delayed food allergies and sensitivities. Once this immune response begins, your body will respond each time you consume the offending food, which further irritates the intestinal lining.

Fortunately, you can reverse leaky gut syndrome and at the same time eliminate delayed food allergies. By following the IBS Program described in this book, you can identify and avoid food allergens. When you avoid these problem foods, your body will have a chance to heal and recover from the damage they have caused. Your intestinal lining will repair itself, and you will experience a marked improvement in your symptoms of IBS.

Try to rotate the foods you eat; eating the same foods day in and day out can contribute to food allergies. In addition, by balancing the intestinal flora and eating an alkaline diet, your body's intestinal lining can be strengthened and brought back to health. (A balanced eating plan is presented in chapter 7.)

NEVER SAY NEVER

If you identify a delayed food allergy, you should eliminate the reactive food from your diet. You will notice an immediate improvement in your IBS symptoms, since your digestive system will no longer be assaulted by the allergenic food. In the coming weeks and months, your digestive system will begin to heal itself, becoming less vulnerable to problem foods. After three months or so, if you want to reintroduce the food, you can do so, provided you have been free of IBS symptoms during the three-month period. Watch for any reactions during the next forty-eight hours.

A true food allergy is a lifelong problem, but many delayed food sensitivities can be cleared up over time. If you remain symptom-free, your body may now be less reactive to this food. Remember, moderation is key; if you overdo it, you may develop the sensitivity again.

On the other hand, if you do react to the food when you try it, avoid it for at least six months before trying to reintroduce it again. Sometimes the long period of digestive rest will allow you to tolerate the food again.

Strike three and you're out. If you reintroduce this same food a third time and continue to react, you can assume that this food is a permanent allergen (even if it does not cause an immediate reaction). Avoid it for life.

Milk intolerance is one of the most common food sensitivities. In my experience, almost all my patients with IBS are milk intolerant. The following chapter discusses this condition in greater detail and provides tips for living with milk intolerance.

Chapter 5

Living with Milk Intolerance

Mother's milk is the ideal nectar for newborns—a complete food replete with the antibodies and nutrients perfectly suited for human growth and development. When babies move from breast or bottle to sippy cup, most well-intentioned mothers introduce cow's milk as the beverage of choice for their children. The dairy industry has done a marvelous job convincing Americans that milk is a healthy beverage, but it is not. Cow's milk is the perfect food for calves, but not for human beings. Milk does not, in fact, do a body good, as advertisers claim. Forget your milk mustache.

One of the first dietary changes I recommend to *all* my patients with IBS is that they eliminate milk and dairy products. I make this blanket recommendation without bothering with diagnostic tests and elimination diets because almost every patient I have ever seen with IBS has been milk intolerant. I don't need to perform the test when I already know what the answer will be.

Some of my patients are skeptical about my recommendation, until they give it a try. I am continually astounded by how often people who eliminate milk and dairy products from their diets have an immediate and dramatic response to this simple change in diet.

Note that I recommend giving up all dairy products, not simply switching to lactose-free products. Grocery store shelves are crowded with lactose-free milk and other products designed for people with lactose intolerance, but these products don't help the many people who have a true sensitivity to milk and dairy products, rather than a simple deficiency in lactase. Someone with a simple lactase deficiency will be able to tolerate dairy products as long as he or she receives supplemental lactase enzymes, but someone who suffers from a broader allergy to "cow"—or a true allergenic response to dairy products—will react to dairy, regardless of the lactase added to the milk.

No doubt, some people with mild lactose intolerance can consume small amounts of lactose-free milk, butter, yogurt, and some cheeses without developing immediate IBS symptoms, but I believe that this chronic exposure to dairy foods weakens the digestive system and leaves the body more vulnerable to food allergies and IBS symptoms. Again, if you have IBS, your best bet is to give up all milk and dairy products completely.

LACTOSE, LACTASE, AND IBS

So what is it about dairy products that sends lactose-intolerant people running to the nearest bathroom? Dairy products contain lactose, a molecule made up of two sugars, glucose and galactose. As part of the digestive process, lactose must be split (or digested) by lactase, an enzyme manufactured in the intestinal lining. When the body lacks sufficient lactase, the lactose is not broken down properly and the complete molecule moves on to the large intestine. As the lactase moves through the digestive system, bacteria cause the sugars to ferment, releasing hydrogen gas and drawing fluid through the intestinal walls into the bowels through the process of osmosis. The result: gas, bloating, cramping, and diarrhea.

Lactose intolerance involves an enzyme deficiency; an allergy to dairy products requires that the body have an antibody response to milk proteins. (For a complete discussion of food allergies, see chapter 4.)

GETTING ENOUGH CALCIUM WITHOUT DAIRY PRODUCTS

Calcium is essential for good health. It helps build strong bones and teeth, helps blood clot, helps nerve and muscle function. If you plan to eliminate dairy products from your diet, increase your consumption of leafy vegetables and other plant-based sources of calcium. You may also want to take supplemental calcium, magnesium, and vitamin D. The recommended daily allowance of calcium is 1,000 milligrams for men, 1,200 for women, and 1,500 for pregnant and lactating women.

Nondairy Sources of Calcium

Broccoli, cooked	2 stalks	530 mg
Sardines (with bones)	2 oz.	240 mg
Collard greens, cooked	6 oz	225 mg
Almonds	3 oz.	210 mg
Soybeans, cooked	6 oz.	150 mg
Tofu	3 oz.	110 mg
Kelp	¼ oz.	80 mg
Sunflower seeds	2 oz.	80 mg
Sesame seeds	2 oz.	75 mg

While many people find it difficult to give up milk-based foods at first, the human body does not need to consume dairy products. Many people believe milk is the ultimate source of calcium, but there are many other more healthful sources of dietary calcium, such as green leafy vegetables. As a matter of fact, milk drinkers tend to have more problems with calcium deficiency than people who consume fewer dairy products. People who eat a balanced overall diet can obtain plenty of calcium from other, healthier foods.

The calcium found in vegetables and fruits has a greater impact on bone health than calcium from dairy products. A study published in *The American Journal of Clinical Nutrition* (2002) found that a high intake of vegetables and fruits had a positive impact on bone health, but dairy did not. Dairy products contain animal proteins, which speed the elimination of calcium from the body and make it more acidic. This can cause calcium to leach from the bones and can cause problems with magnesium absorption, leading to osteoporosis. In addition, we absorb only 30 percent of the calcium found in milk, compared to 40 to 70 percent of the calcium found in vegetables and fruits. An eight-ounce glass of calcium-fortified orange juice has the same amount of calcium as an eight-ounce glass of milk, but you would absorb more calcium by drinking the juice than you would from the milk. Better yet: Eat whole oranges, which provide the calcium without the increased sugar load.

WHO DEVELOPS LACTOSE INTOLERANCE?

Lactose intolerance is the most common digestive disorder in the world. In fact, with the exception of people from Northern Europe, most adults worldwide have some difficulty digesting dairy products.

A person's ability to metabolize lactose changes throughout his or her lifetime. Almost all babies are born with high levels of lactase enzyme in their intestines. Within a year or two, levels of the enzyme begin to drop off in children with an inherited predisposition to lactose intolerance. During adulthood, many people lose the ability to manufacture lactase. Fully 70 to 80 percent of all African Americans, Native Americans, Jews, and Asians worldwide experience lactose intolerance by the time they reach adulthood.

Some people do not realize they have lactose intolerance. They may have noticed some minor symptoms that come and go depending on diet, but they may have grown accustomed to the fairly mild symptoms. These people may have lower levels of lactase in their systems than they once did, but they still have enough to handle the challenges presented by occasional dairy foods since most adults do not drink milk by the glass. In other words, they can handle a small bowl of cereal with milk in the morning, but an ice cream sundae can send them over the edge.

MORE REASONS TO FORGET THE MILK MUSTACHE

Suffering from IBS is reason enough to give up dairy products, but there are other reasons as well. Cow's milk contains proteins that are difficult for humans to digest; when these undigested proteins enter the lower digestive system, they putrefy and cause digestive problems. Dairy products encourage the production of excess mucus in the body, burdening the respiratory, digestive, and immune systems. Not surprisingly, when my patients give up dairy products, they often experience markedly fewer colds and sinus infections.

In addition, milk is often contaminated with low levels of pesticides, antibiotics, and other chemicals. Dairy farmers routinely inject their cows with recombinant bovine growth hormone (rBGH), a genetically engineered drug designed to increase milk production by 10 to 25 percent. This synthetic hormone passes on to humans through the cow's milk; milk containing rBGH also contains high levels of insulin growth factor, which has been linked to breast and colon cancer, juvenile diabetes, hypertension, and glucose intolerance.

Milk has also been linked to prostate cancer. An eleven-year study of nearly twenty-one thousand men published in *The American Journal of Clinical Nutrition* (2001) found that men who consumed more than 600 milligrams of calcium from dairy products daily had a 32 percent increased risk of developing prostate cancer compared to men who consumed only 150 milligrams of calcium from dairy. (To give you an idea of how much milk that is, a six-ounce glass of milk contains 225 milligrams of calcium.)

Ironically, milk consumption has also been linked to an increased risk of hip fracture in women. According to the Harvard University Nurses Health Study, which followed seventy-eight thousand women for twelve years, the women who consumed the highest levels of calcium in the form of dairy products had more broken bones than women who rarely drank milk. In addition, a woman's risk of hip fractures increased in relation to her increased consumption of dairy products. While the exact cause of this link has not been confirmed, some researchers believe that the high protein content of milk pushes the body into a negative calcium balance because the calcium is used in the metabolism of the protein. Other researchers speculate that high dairy consumption alters bone metabolism by overusing and damaging the osteoblasts, specialized cells that help the bones absorb calcium. In any case, the evidence suggests that high consumption of dairy products weakens the bones.

SUBSTITUTES: WHEN YOU CAN'T HAVE DAIRY

If you like the taste and texture of dairy foods, you can be creative by switching to dairylike food substitutes. The following are some creative ways you can utilize alternatives to traditional milk products:

- Instead of cow's milk, use nut milks, Lassi (water and rose water), rice milk, and soy milk.
- Instead of butter, use clarified butter (ghee) or homemade

clarified butter; see the recipe on page 109. (The whey is removed, making clarified butter less allergenic than regular butter.)

- Instead of milk or cream in baked recipes, use water, fruit juice, or even vegetable stock (this is especially good in breads).
- Instead of using milk in cream sauces and custards, choose nut milk, almond milk, or Rice Dream beverage. All can be used freely in cooking and maintain the texture and rich flavor associated with creamed sauces.
- Instead of ricotta cheese, cottage cheese, yogurt, or sour cream, use feta, Romano, or goat cheese when cooking.

Dairy-Free Cookbooks

Some cooks enjoy the challenge of adapting recipes to a dairy-free diet, while others prefer recipes designed with the lactose intolerant in mind. The following books can help you prepare dishes that are both dairy-free and delicious:

- *Dairy-Free Cookbook,* second edition, by Jane Zukin (Prima, 1998)
- *The Lactose-Free Cookbook* by Sheri Updike (Warner, 1998)
- *Totally Dairy-Free Cooking* by Louis Lanza and Laura Morton (William Morrow, 2000)
- *The Uncheese Cookbook: Creating Amazing Dairy-Free Cheese Substitutes and Classic "Uncheese" Dishes* by Joanne Stepaniak (Book Pub, 1994)

Make Your Own Nut Milk

1 cup raw almonds or almond meal (ground almonds)
1 quart water
1 tablespoon cold-pressed oil, melted ghee, or clarified butter

Blanch the almonds by pouring boiling water over them. After 1 minute, slip the skins off with your fingers. Blend all the ingredients in a blender until smooth (about 3 minutes). Strain and drink.

If you prefer, you can use other nuts or combinations. Suggestions: almond-coconut milk (using equal parts almonds and raw or flaked unsweetened coconut), almond-cashew milk (using equal parts almonds and cashews), almond-sesame milk (using equal parts almonds and hulled sesame seeds).

Where Is the Milk?

Dairy products can be found in a number of unexpected places. The following products contain milk or other ingredients that can irritate people with lactose intolerance:

- Baked goods: Breads, bagels, rolls, biscuits, crackers, cookies, cakes, pies.
- Sweets: Candy, ice cream, chocolate.
- Miscellaneous: Creamed vegetables and soups, luncheon meats, quiche, pasta, salad dressings, sauces, and yogurt.

Chapter 6

Candidiasis, or Yeast Overgrowth

Ask people what they think of when they hear the word *yeast* and most would describe aromatic loaves of freshly baked bread. Ask doctors who treat IBS what they think of when they hear the same word and the answer probably would be candidiasis, or yeast overgrowth.

If you have IBS, you almost certainly have an overgrowth of the yeast known as *Candida albicans* throughout your digestive system. Candida is one of more than six hundred different types of yeast that live in the gastrointestinal system—the mouth, throat, stomach, intestines, and genitourinary tracts. When you are healthy, *C. albicans* lives in harmony with other yeasts and with acidophilus, the "good bacteria" that help keep the flora in balance. Under certain circumstances, however, this yeast will multiply and overwhelm the healthy flora. The result is a condition known as candidiasis.

Left untreated, the yeast continues to reproduce, developing rhizoids, or roots, that grow into the intestinal wall or other mucous linings. Once the yeast is implanted, *C. albicans* poisons the bloodstream with mycotoxins (from the Latin words *myco,* meaning "fungus," and *toxin,* meaning "poison") caused by the fermentation of glucose, proteins, and fats. The intestinal membranes swell and become inflamed as the germs invade deeper into the tissues. The body makes antibodies to *C. albicans* organism, leading to a hypersensitivity reaction, which further compromises the system and makes the body more sensitive to yeast. As a result, you can develop nose, throat, sinus, ear, bronchial, bladder, and other infections as well as additional food sensitivities and symptoms of IBS.

HOW YEAST OVERGROWTH DEVELOPS

In order for yeast to grow out of control, the digestive environment must be compromised in some way. The following are common problems that contribute to yeast overgrowth:

- **The level of hydrochloric acid in the stomach falls too low.** If the level of gastric juices—including hydrochloric acid, pancreatic enzymes, and bile—drops too low, yeast can flourish. As mentioned earlier, the use of medications such as Tagamet, Zantac, Prilosec, and other drugs to inhibit the production of hydrochloric acid can make yeast overgrowth worse. In addition, low levels of hydrochloric acid can result in a number of other symptoms, including bloating, belching, flatulence, indigestion, diarrhea or constipation, multiple food allergies, rectal itching, iron deficiency, intestinal parasites, *Helicobacter pylori,* undigested food in the stool, and upper digestive tract gassiness. For this reason, I do not recommend the use of antacids for the treatment of IBS or candidiasis.

• **The body's pH becomes too acidic.** The pH inside the stomach should be slightly acidic, but inside the small intestine and in the blood and urine, it should be slightly basic. This pH level must be kept within a fairly tight range to encourage the growth of probiotic or "good" bacteria. When the body is too acidic, the friendly bacteria that normally metabolize and control sugars cannot thrive, allowing the yeast to feast on the excess sugar. As the yeast multiplies, it produces increasing amounts of acidic waste, which makes the environment still more acidic and hospitable to the yeast. To break the synergistic relationship between acid and yeast, you must increase the body's pH or alkalinize your tissues. This can be accomplished through changes in diet (see chapter 7) and the use of appropriate supplements (see chapter 11).

• **Low levels of pancreatic enzymes cause poor digestion.** Incomplete digestion of foods, especially proteins, contributes to yeast overgrowth and IBS. When foods are not adequately broken down by the pancreatic enzymes, they are consumed by harmful bacteria that release toxins as they digest the food. In a healthy digestive system, the pancreas produces enzymes that include lipases (to digest fats), proteases (to break protein into single amino acids), and amylases (to break starch into smaller sugars). These enzymes are also essential in keeping the small intestine free of yeast and other parasites.

• **A diet filled with sugar and alcoholic beverages contributes to yeast overgrowth.** Alcohol is broken down into sugar in the digestive process. This or any other sugar literally feeds the yeast, allowing it to grow with vigor.

• **Use of antibiotics, especially broad-spectrum antibiotics, kills helpful bacteria.** Antibiotics such as ampicillin, penicillin, and cephalosporin kill not only the harmful bacteria, but the helpful bacteria as well. Problems also arise when a patient is on long-term antibiotics, such as tetracycline for acne. When the digestive system is out of balance, the stage is set for yeast to grow out of control.

• **Use of birth control pills encourages yeast overgrowth.** The hormones in birth control pills stimulate the growth of yeast by raising the amount of sugar (glycogen) in the vagina. For the same reasons, the hormonal changes associated with pregnancy, the menstrual cycle, or menopause can also cause yeast overgrowth. While a number of factors contribute to a woman's decision on what form of birth control to use, a woman with yeast problems may want to choose another form of contraception.

• **Use of immunosuppressant drugs compromises the immune system.** Cortisone, prednisone, other steroids, and chemotherapy drugs suppress the immune system, leaving the body more susceptible to yeast overgrowth. Of course, there are times that these medicines are necessary, but in these cases patients should be sure to follow the dietary guidelines and take the supplements recommended later in the book.

The Problem with Carbohydrates

When you consume simple carbohydrates—such as refined sugar, brown sugar, corn syrup, white rice, white bread, white pasta, and white flour—they are converted into glucose, which feeds yeast and creates rapid shifts in blood sugar levels. When you eat a lot of sugary foods, your pancreas tends to overreact and release too much insulin. This causes your blood glucose to drop rapidly, often lower than it was before you ate anything. When this happens, you're apt to feel nervous, tired, and hungry. In response, you crave sweets and additional simple carbohydrates. As soon as you eat them, you feel better temporarily, then the blood sugar repeats the up-and-down cycle. These simple sugars feed the yeast as well.

DO YOU HAVE YEAST OVERGROWTH?

As part of my regular screening for IBS, I ask my patients a series of questions to evaluate the extent of yeast overgrowth. (I assume that the patient has candidiasis, since almost every patient I have ever seen with IBS has had yeast overgrowth as well.) The classic telltale signs include a white tongue (thrush), toenail or fingernail fungus, vaginal yeast infections, and jock itch or athlete's foot. (*Candida albicans* comes from a Latin phrase meaning "glowing white," and it was so named because this yeast is white in color.)

Overgrowth of yeast can affect virtually every system of the body, with the gastrointestinal, genitourinary, endocrine, nervous, and immune systems being the most susceptible. Common symptoms of candidiasis include:

- Digestive disorders, including IBS
- Gastrointestinal symptoms: thrush, bloating, gas, rectal itching
- Vaginal yeast infection
- Urinary tract infections
- Athlete's foot or jock itch
- Fungal toenails or fingernails
- Cravings for sugar, bread, or alcohol
- Diaper rash
- Fatigue
- Irritability (especially when hungry)
- Premenstrual syndrome and menstrual problems
- Fibromyalgia
- Headaches
- Brain fog
- Skin problems or itching
- Numbness or tingling in the extremities
- Respiratory problems
- Depression
- Hypoglycemia
- Short attention span
- Loss of libido

Symptoms often become worse in damp or moldy places, or after consumption of foods containing yeast or sugar. In someone with a severely compromised immune system (such as advanced cancer or AIDS), the yeast overgrowth can spread throughout the body, causing a condition known as systemic candidiasis. In the most severe cases, candida can travel through the bloodstream to invade every organ of the body, causing a life-threatening type of blood poisoning known as candida septicemia.

To confirm a suspected case of candidiasis, you can measure the *C. albicans* antibody levels in the blood or conduct a stool analysis test. A comprehensive digestive stool analysis provides a great deal of additional information on digestive function, the intestinal environment, and nutrient absorption. (Laboratories that provide a complete stool analysis include Great Smokies Diagnostic Laboratory, 800-522-4762; National BioTech Laboratory, 800-846-6285; Diagnos-Techs, 800-87-TESTS; and Meridian Valley Laboratory, 253-859-8700.)

Instead of getting bogged down with testing, I recommend that all my IBS patients assume they have a problem with yeast and follow the IBS diet listed in chapter 7. If you follow the program for thirty days, yeast will be minimized or brought back into balance.

A Special Word to Nursing Mothers

If a breast-fed baby develops oral thrush or a nursing mother develops a thrush infection of the nipples, both mother and baby should be treated to eradicate the infection, even if only one of them seems to be affected. If mother and child are not treated together, they may continually reinfect one another. In babies, oral thrush may look like tiny milk drops in the mouth.

THE GOOD NEWS

Candidiasis almost never occurs in people with healthy immune systems who eat a diet low in sugar and yeast. This book can help you get your yeast under control by changing your diet.

When conventional doctors diagnose candidiasis, they often turn to medications again. Commonly prescribed antifungal medications include nystatin, Diflucan (fluconazole), miconazole, and Nizoral (ketoconazole). Some of these medications can be toxic to the liver. In addition, the prescribe-and-medicate approach to treating the symptoms does not address the underlying problem that caused yeast overgrowth in the first place.

Instead of turning to medications, you should create an environment that is inhospitable to yeast. I often tell my patients to imagine that having yeast overgrowth is similar to having pests in your kitchen. If your kitchen is overrun with bugs, you don't have to use pesticides to kill the bugs. You could get rid of the garbage and open food in the room, and the bugs will leave when there is nothing for them to eat. The same is true of controlling yeast: You don't need to use medications to kill the yeast; simply eliminate the food source for the yeast, and they will disappear on their own. If you normalize the bacterial flora in the gastrointestinal tract, you don't need drugs in most cases.

TREATING CANDIDIASIS WITH DIET

The foods you eat can either feed the yeast and encourage it to thrive—or starve the yeast into submission. The following guidelines can help you tame the yeast in your digestive system. Specific food plans are discussed in chapter 7.

Foods to Avoid

- Sugars of any kind, including corn syrup, sugarcane, beets, dates, maple syrup, honey, molasses, fructose, dextrose, maltose, lactose, and fruit juices.
- Artificial sweeteners.
- Foods containing brewer's yeast—used in alcoholic beverages, including beer, wine, champagne, brandy, whiskey, rum, ciders, and root beer.
- Foods containing baker's yeast—used in baked goods, breads, rolls, and pastries.
- Mushrooms.
- Fruits and vegetables with any sign of mold growth on them. In severe cases, fruits of all kinds should be avoided for thirty days because they are readily converted to simple sugars, which feed the yeast.
- Fermented beverages and condiments, including cider, ketchup, mayonnaise, pickled vegetables, pickles, salad dressings (use lemon and olive oil instead), soy sauce, and vinegar.
- Cheeses. Avoid all types of hard cheeses, which are a good source of mold.
- Processed and smoked meats and fish, including hot dogs, sausages, luncheon meats, corned beef, salami, smoked salmon, ham, and pastrami. These are processed with sugar, spices, yeast, and other preservatives.
- Canned, bottled, or frozen fruit and vegetable juices. Juices contain lots of sugar, and they are commonly made from

overripened or damaged produce; generally the skin of the fruit contains surface mold and rotten spots, which are pulverized into the juice.

- Dried fruits.
- Coffee and tea. Caffeine can aggravate yeast overgrowth. In addition, teas made from dried leaves, pods, and flowering plants tend to accumulate mold on them.
- Melons. Cantaloupes and other melons tend to develop molds and should be avoided.
- Alcoholic beverages of any kind.

Foods You Can Eat

The following foods generally do not contribute to yeast growth. You can eat them freely, unless you have determined that you have a sensitivity or allergy to them.

- **Vegetables and legumes:** Artichokes, asparagus, beans (all kinds), broccoli, brussels sprouts, cabbage, carrots, cauliflower, celery, cucumbers, eggplant, garlic, green beans, greens (beet, chard, collard, kale), kohlrabi, leeks, lettuce, okra, onions, parsley, parsnips, peas, peppers (all kinds), plantains, potatoes (white and sweet), pumpkin, radishes, rutabagas, scallions, soybeans, spinach, sprouts, squash (all kinds), tofu, tomatoes, turnips, and yams.

- **Nuts:** Almonds, Brazil nuts, filberts, macadamias, pecans, pine nuts, and walnuts.

- **Seeds:** Flaxseed, pumpkin, sesame, and sunflower.

- **Fish:** Cod, crab, halibut, salmon, shrimp, trout, tuna, and other fresh fish.

• **Red meats:** Beef, buffalo, lamb, pork (uncured and unsmoked only), rabbit, veal, venison, and other red meats.

• **Butters:** Almond and other nut butters (except peanut), sesame, and sunflower.

• **Whole grains:** Barley, corn, millet, oat, brown rice, rye, spelt, teff, wheat, and wild rice.

• **Nongrains:** Amaranth, buckwheat, quinoa, arrowroot, and tapioca.

• **Poultry:** Chicken, Cornish hen, duck, eggs, goose, pheasant, turkey, other poultry.

• **Beverages:** Water, sparkling water, lemon or lime water.

• **Fats:** Butter, ghee, oils (cold-pressed, unrefined), olive oil, and flaxseed oil. Avoid peanut oil.

• **Fresh fruits:** Avoid for the first thirty days; after this, you may have low-carbohydrate fruits on the list on pages 87–88.

Chapter 7

How to Customize Your Diet to Beat IBS

For people with IBS, eating can be a source of great anxiety. Will you pay for that hot fudge sundae with an agonizing evening of cramping and diarrhea? Will the hamburger you ate at the company picnic send you home doubled over in pain? Once the symptoms start, IBS sufferers often wonder which food brought them on. Was it the ice cream or the chocolate sauce, the hamburger or the bun?

In the simplest terms, to avoid the symptoms of IBS, you must know which foods to eliminate from your diet. This can be a daunting task, especially since most of the foods we eat contain a wide range of ingredients and additives. But there is good news: You will be able to end your suffering with IBS and enjoy food again by following the IBS Eating Plan described in this chapter. This plan will help you regain balance in your digestive system, identify which foods trigger food sensitivities, and develop a lifelong plan for balanced eating.

Of course, changing your eating habits isn't easy, but the IBS Eating Plan offers the best possible reward for compliance—you will experience relief from your IBS symptoms. Your days of suffering will soon be over; in my experience, most people note significant relief from IBS within the first thirty days, and many feel markedly better within the first week!

EASY AS A, B, C, AND D

You can cure your IBS by changing your diet and nourishing your body with appropriate nutritional supplements. The IBS Eating Plan I have designed is as easy as A, B, C, and D:

A: Accentuate the Alkaline
B: Banish Bread (and other yeast foods)
C: Cut Carbohydrates
D: Drop Dairy from Your Diet

By changing your diet to reflect these core principles, you will reach the appropriate pH level both in your digestive system and throughout your body; prevent the ravages of yeast overgrowth; avoid simple carbohydrates that contribute to weight gain and poor food choices; and avoid dairy foods, which are among the most allergenic of the foods we eat.

In addition, the IBS Eating Plan will help you identify the allergenic foods that may be contributing to your IBS symptoms. By starting with less allergenic foods at the beginning of the diet and adding foods to the meal plan over a span of several weeks (or months, depending on your situation), you will be able to determine which foods may be causing delayed food sensitivities and contributing to your IBS.

UNDERSTANDING THE CORE PRINCIPLES

The IBS Eating Plan is a synthesis of the issues discussed throughout the book. The program builds on several basic principles:

Principle A: Accentuate the alkaline by increasing your consumption of high-protein, low-carbohydrate foods. As discussed on page 18, the foods you eat affect the pH levels of your digestive system, your blood, and your entire body. Simply put, foods are classified as either alkaline or acidic, based not on how they taste but on the residue left after they have been metabolized in the body. People with IBS need to eat a more alkaline diet, which includes moderate amounts of protein and some low-sugar complex carbohydrates. Fortunately, this approach to eating fits well with many of the other aspects of a healthy diet.

Principle B: Banish breads (and other yeasty foods). As discussed in detail in chapter 6, yeast overgrowth is very common among people with IBS. Eliminating sugar and yeast from the diet can help to reduce yeast overgrowth inside the digestive tract. The yeast found in foods (such as brewer's yeast and baker's yeast), as well as molds found on certain foods (such as hard cheese and aging foods), are "cousins" to *C. albicans* and can contribute to candidiasis.

Principle C: Cut carbohydrates. As discussed in chapter 6, simple carbohydrates stimulate the growth of yeast and contribute to IBS. You should choose high-protein foods that are low in carbohydrates.

Principle D: Drop dairy from your diet. As discussed in detail in chapter 5, most people with IBS also suffer from milk and dairy intolerance. If you have milk hypersensitivity, consuming dairy products will irritate and inflame the digestive tract, altering the environment of the gastrointestinal tract. I recommend that you avoid dairy products entirely.

As you work through the diet plan, you will reintroduce potential problem foods one at a time. Once your digestive system regains balance, you can experiment with expanding the foods in your diet. You should add potential problem foods back one at a time, while watching to see if you have an adverse reaction to a food when you begin eating it again. As you gradually expand the foods in your Core Diet, you will be able to determine precisely which ones you can include in your diet and which are best left on your plate.

PHASES IN THE IBS EATING PLAN

As is true with most diet programs, the IBS Eating Plan introduces dietary changes in phases. Your diet will change over time as your digestive system repairs itself.

Phase 1: Healing and Repair with the Core Foods (1 to 2 Weeks)

The goal of Phase 1 is for you to heal and stabilize your digestive system by consuming a predominantly alkaline diet. During Phase 1, you may eat as much as you like of the foods listed as part of the Core Diet on page 81 This is not a weight-loss diet, but many of my patients lose weight because they are eating healthier and more satisfying foods.

Strive to consume only whole, unprocessed foods (organic, if possible), and prepare them yourself. (The menu plans in chapter 8 may be of assistance.) Avoid commercially prepared foods, which often contain additives and preservatives. Keep your diet simple, so that you will be able to identify any foods that may be triggering your IBS symptoms.

In the first few days on the program, many patients experience immediate improvement in their IBS symptoms. At the same time, however, some people report that they feel tired, anxious, and irritable, which may be an ongoing reaction to foods eaten earlier in the day; or the body may be responding to the detoxification or a candida die-off reaction. In the coming weeks, you will feel much better as your body heals and stabilizes.

Keep a detailed food journal, listing every food you eat, when you eat it, and how you feel throughout the day. This journal will help you identify possible food allergens and patterns in your reactions to certain foods. (A sample food journal is included in chapter 12.)

You should not move on to Phase 2 until you feel better and experience some relief from your IBS symptoms. Most people will be able to enter Phase 2 within two weeks, but it may take longer for some IBS sufferers. If your IBS symptoms continue after three weeks in Phase 1, consider following the liquid-only diet described on page 92 to cleanse the system, then adding alkaline foods gradually to identify possible allergenic foods. In addition, you may want to visit a doctor and undergo blood tests to determine if some of the foods in the Core Diet may be triggering a reaction. (For more information on allergy testing, see chapter 3.)

Phase 2: Reintroducing Foods One at a Time (3 Weeks to 3 Months)

During the next phase of your diet, you will begin adding foods one at a time. You can begin to add grains, then add other foods as you wish. After each new food is added, wait a day or two before adding another so that you can identify any foods that are causing allergic reactions. (See chapter 4 for additional information on recognizing the symptoms of a food sensitivity or allergy.) Continue to keep a food journal to help you identify allergic reactions.

If you experience IBS symptoms after adding a food, eliminate it from your diet and put it on a list of foods not to eat. Once your body has regained stability, begin trying new foods once again.

In addition, be sure to rotate your foods to minimize your risk of allergic reaction. Eating the same food day after day increases the likelihood of having an adverse reaction to it. Instead, limit foods that do not appear on the Core Diet to once a week.

Phase 3: Maintenance (Lifetime)

When you reach a state of balance and improved digestive health, your body can tolerate a somewhat less alkaline diet. The basic plan should become your healthy eating plan for a lifetime, but *occasionally* you can indulge in decadent foods that are not part of your Core Diet. In other words, if you crave fresh corn on the cob with butter, a blueberry muffin fresh from the oven, or even an ice cream sundae, you can probably tolerate these guilty pleasures every once in a while.

I recommend that you "cheat" on the program no more than once or twice a month to minimize your risk of weakening your digestive system and developing IBS symptoms again. Our bodies are very resilient; we have many built-in systems to buffer the damage we do to ourselves every day. That being said, when you use up your reserves, you will feel the same digestive problems you are working to eliminate. It's similar to the shock absorbers in your car. When you have good shock absorbers, you can go over a bump and not feel a thing. But when the shock absorbers are shot, you'll feel every pebble.

The same phenomenon applies to IBS. Your digestive system has quite a few compensatory mechanisms. When you get rid of the stresses that weaken your body, you can strengthen your system and tolerate the occasional variation in diet. This does not mean you will be able to eat allergenic foods or that you can revert to your old, harmful ways of eating without expecting the same problems to resurface. It does mean that you live in the real world and will encounter dietary temptations on an ongoing basis. The occasional dietary misstep should not be a big step backward. If you do have a strong reaction to a problem food, eliminate the food from your diet and allow the experience to serve as a strong reminder that your diet was working.

THE CORE DIET: FOODS TO CHOOSE

Your goal should be to eat a large variety of different foods and rotate them often to minimize the risk of developing food sensitivities. (The more often you eat a particular food, the more likely you are to develop an allergy or sensitivity to it.) You should strive to consume foods that are alkaline, low in carbohydrates, and high in protein. Use the following charts as a guide for choosing the foods in the Core Diet.

Meat, Fish, Shellfish, and Fowl

These foods are excellent sources of protein. Consume six to eight ounces of protein throughout the day. (You can eat more, if needed, during the first few weeks as you adjust to the new diet.)

- **Fish:** Freshwater and saltwater fish are excellent sources of high-grade protein and essential polyunsaturated fatty acids. Fresh fish is preferable, but canned tuna, salmon, and sardines are acceptable. Canned fish should be packed in water and carefully drained.

- **Shellfish:** If you are allergic to shellfish, do not include these foods in your diet. Shellfish is also an excellent source of protein.

- **Fowl:** Turkey, Cornish game hen, goose, chicken, squab, pheasant, and duck are all excellent sources of protein. Duck and goose are high in fat, especially near the skin. If you have a weight problem, skin should be removed before cooking.

- **Meat:** Conventional meats—steaks, roasts, chops, and so forth—are also high-quality protein, but they tend to be high in fat. Buy lean meat; choose products labeled "good" rather than "choice" or "prime." Muscle meat should be trimmed of all visible fat before cooking; it should be cooked on a rack so that the fat released during the cooking process drips out and the meat does not stew in its juices. Gravies should be skimmed of fat. Do not consume muscle meat more than three times per week, and limit serving size to four ounces.

NOTE: *Canned meat, cold cuts, hot dogs, sausages, and pork are not permitted.*

Dairy

- **Eggs:** Eggs are an excellent source of complete protein.
- **Butter:** Unsalted butter is acceptable. Quantities should be limited if you have concerns about weight.
- **Goat's milk:** This milk is acceptable; cow's milk is not.

NOTE: *Cow's milk and other dairy products made with milk should be avoided.*

Nuts and Seeds

These are a good source of protein. Servings should be restricted to two tablespoons. They should be eaten fresh from the shell, not roasted or salted. They are listed in order of overall value to the diet; those not listed are not permitted:

- Pignolias
- Brazil nuts
- Pumpkin or squash kernels
- Sesame
- Almonds
- Walnuts (black and English)
- Pecans

- Toasted soybeans
- Sunflower seeds
- Hazelnuts (filberts)

NOTE: *Peanuts are not permitted.*

Vegetables

You may have unlimited quantities of the lowest-sugar (3 percent carbohydrate) and lower-sugar (6 percent carbohydrate) vegetables; limit the quantity of low-sugar (10 percent carbohydrate) vegetables to half a cup per day. Other vegetables are not part of the Core Diet; they should be added in Phase 2 and consumed no more than once per week, if you do not experience a reaction to them.

Lowest-Sugar Vegetables (3 Percent Carbohydrate)

- Bean sprouts
- Beet greens
- Celery
- Chicory
- Chinese cabbage
- Chives
- Cucumbers
- Endive
- Escarole
- Fennel
- Lettuce
- Olives
- Parsley

- Dill and sour pickles
- Poke
- Radishes
- Rhubarb, raw
- Watercress

Lower-Sugar Vegetables (6 Percent Carbohydrate)

- Asparagus
- Bamboo shoots
- Broccoli
- Cabbage, raw
- Cauliflower
- Chard
- Collard greens, raw
- Dandelion greens
- Eggplant
- Kale
- Leeks
- Mustard greens
- Okra
- Green onions
- Peppers
- Rhubarb, cooked
- Sauerkraut
- Spinach
- Turnips
- Turnip greens
- Water chestnuts
- Zucchini

Low-Sugar Vegetables (10 Percent Carbohydrate)

- Artichokes
- Green beans, French or wax
- Carrots
- Celeriac
- Cabbage, cooked
- Brussels sprouts
- Collard greens, cooked
- Chervil
- Garden cress
- Kohlrabi
- Onion, raw
- Rutabaga
- Tomato

NOTE: *Corn, potatoes, sweet pickles, sweet potatoes, and yams are not permitted.*

Grains

Grains should be eliminated from the diet during Phase 1. (Vegans who feel they need to include grains in Phase 1 can include brown rice, quinoa, and amaranth on the list.) Once your IBS symptoms have been eliminated, you can begin to add grains one at a time, in the following order:

- Brown rice
- Quinoa
- Amaranth
- Oatmeal

- Rye
- Buckwheat (kasha)
- Millet
- Wheat
- Barley
- Flaxseed
- Rice

NOTE: *White bread, crackers, macaroni, spaghetti, pancakes, rolls, waffles, and products made with refined flour are not permitted.*

Fruits

Fresh fruits are an excellent source of vitamins and minerals. They can be used to replace high-carbohydrate foods such as candy, cookies, and cakes, which contain few nutrients and should be avoided. The list of acceptable fruits is divided into three categories: lowest-sugar (7 percent carbohydrate), lower-sugar (10 percent carbohydrate), and low-sugar (15 percent carbohydrate). You may have unlimited quantities of the lowest- and lower-sugar fruits, but limit low-sugar fruits to one serving per day. Other fruits are not part of the Core Diet; they should be added in Phase 2 and consumed no more than once per week, if you do not experience a reaction to them. Watch citrus fruits and melons for intolerance; choose only whole fruits, not juices.

Lowest-Sugar Fruits (7 Percent Carbohydrate)

- Avocado

- Watermelon
- Rhubarb

Lower-Sugar Fruits (10 Percent Carbohydrate)

- Boysenberries
- Cantaloupe
- Casaba melon
- Coconut, fresh only
- Cranberries, raw
- Fruit salad (no grapes)
- Gooseberries
- Honeydew melon
- Lemon
- Lime
- Muskmelon
- Strawberries

Low-Sugar Fruits (15 Percent Carbohydrate)

- Apples—1 small
- Apricots—1 small
- Blackberries—½ cup
- Cherries—½ cup
- Dewberries—½ cup
- Elderberries—½ cup
- Grapefruit—½ large
- Grapefruit juice—½ cup
- Loganberries—½ cup
- Oranges—1 small
- Orange juice—½ cup

- Peaches—1 small
- Pears—1 average
- Pineapple—2 slices
- Plums—2 small
- Raspberries—½ cup
- Tangerines—1 average
- Youngberries—½ cup

NOTE: *Bananas, grapes, mangos, dried fruits, and fruits canned in syrup are not permitted.*

Beverages

- Springwater
- Herbal teas and decaffeinated coffees
- Ginger tea (half a teaspoon of gingerroot steeped in hot water and strained)

NOTE: *Colored plastic bottles should be avoided; clear is okay. Tap water should be avoided, unless you have a reverse-osmosis water filter. No alcoholic beverages, caffeine, cocoa, coffee, cola, or soft drinks are permitted.*

Condiments

You may make your own condiments from fresh herbs, spices, polyunsaturated oils, vinegar, and lemon juice. Use oils that are cold-pressed. Sweet 'N Low and NutraSweet are not permitted; Splenda and stevia are acceptable, but not recommended. Dextrose, fructose, glucose, hexitol, lactose, maltose, manitol, sorbitol, and sucrose are all forms of sugar and are not allowed in the form of a sweetener; they are acceptable in limited amounts as part of a natural whole food.

Fats

Fats are permitted in limited amounts. We need some essential fatty acids because the body cannot produce them itself. One tablespoon a day of safflower or sesame oil is enough to meet the requirement. Excess fat is not good for you. Do not use margarine.

GENERAL GUIDELINES FOR HEALTHY EATING

Many of my patients with IBS fear food. They know that if they consume the wrong foods, they will pay with hours of cramping, bloating, and pain. There is no need for anxiety about eating; instead, you need to learn the basic rules of healthy eating. Beyond food selection, the following tips can help you minimize your IBS:

- Chew your food thoroughly. The digestive process begins in your mouth; give your saliva a chance to do its job. When poorly chewed food particles make their way into the digestive system, the bacteria in your gut have a feast, releasing gas, which can cause problems with cramping, bloating, and flatulence.
- Drink at least six to eight glasses of pure water per day. Water is essential to all cellular functions and for the removal of waste and toxic products from the body. (If you have any cardiac problems that require fluid restriction, notify your doctor prior to increasing any fluids.)

- Limit fluid intake during meals; it dilutes the stomach acid. Keep a water bottle with you and sip throughout the day.
- Eat three meals and three balanced snacks per day. I highly recommend that you have regular meals at regular times. Don't leave the house without eating breakfast. If you need to snack between meals, raw vegetables, nuts, or seeds are great for fighting hunger pangs and avoiding fluctuations in blood sugar, which can trigger binge eating.
- Do not overeat. Consuming large quantities at a single meal stresses the digestive system.
- When you eat meat or poultry, choose brands that do not use growth hormones or antibiotics, which can alter the hormone levels in the body and stress the immune system. Choose organic, free-range meat and poultry when possible.
- Whenever possible, buy fruits and vegetables that are certified organic. Organic foods should have less pesticide residue than nonorganic products. Look for the U.S. Department of Agriculture's "organic" label, which recently replaced the private certification network that was in place before 1998.
- Restrict salt intake. Use sea salt or mineral salt rather than iodized salt, which is deficient in many minerals.
- Eliminate foods that contain chemical additives. Avoid foods containing margarine, MSG (monosodium glutamate), NutraSweet, saccharin, aspartame, olestra, hydrolyzed protein, and sodium caseinate. These additives can be toxic to the liver, and they stress the immune system. In addition, when aspartame breaks down in the body, it releases a type of alcohol called methanol. Large

doses of aspartame can change the ratio of amino acids in the bloodstream, which in turn disturbs various neurotransmitters, acting as a neurotoxin.

- Do not consume alcohol, which is converted into sugar in the body and can exacerbate yeast overgrowth.
- Become an educated consumer; take time to read food and beverage labeling.

Cleansing with a Liquid-Only Diet

If your IBS symptoms continue after two weeks of following the Phase 1 plan, consider cleaning your system with a liquid-only fast. The liquid diet is intended as a periodic rest for the intestines; you may want to opt for one day of fasting every week or so to refresh your digestive system. A liquid-only diet is not a juice fast, and it does not involve a restriction in caloric intake. I recommend that you consume at least one eight-ounce glass of the following beverages each hour, but you can drink more if you need to in order to feel satisfied. Your goal should be to consume three or more quarts of fluid during the day. Choose from the following beverages:

- **Miso broth** (preferably with hatcho miso, aged more than twenty-four months) is a fully fermented product derived from soy; it is easily digested. Miso, available at health food stores, rarely causes allergic reactions, even for those with soy, yeast, or mold sensitivities.

- **Watermelon juice** is a surprisingly tasty drink made from blended ripe watermelon pieces (without seeds). A small amount of ginger tea or compatible liquid can be added to start the blending process. Watermelon juice can be prepared in the morning and stored, covered, in the refrigerator for use during the day. (The juice should be covered to prevent air from oxidizing the fruit and reducing the nutritional quality.)

- **Ginger tea** should be made from whole fresh gingerroot (available in most grocery produce areas). The best gingerroot currently comes from Hawaii. To make ginger tea, peel and then freeze the fresh ginger, thaw until it is soft, slice and dice the juicy root, and steep a tablespoon of it in a warmed pot of hot water for ten minutes. Ginger tea is tasty at any temperature and can be refrigerated for several days in a tightly sealed jar.

- **Vegetable juice** is an outstanding source of minerals, especially calcium, magnesium, potassium, and zinc. Be sure to choose only organic vegetables since many vegetables, especially root vegetables, will absorb and concentrate the chemicals in the soil, including pesticides, fungicides, and other toxins. Carrot juice is the staple of vegetable juices, but because of its high carbohydrate content it should be used in combination with other vegetables. Try mixing carrot juice with equal parts of parsley, celery, spinach, artichokes, beets, beet greens, watercress, cilantro, cabbage, or other green leafy vegetables. Change the proportions or dilute the juice to suit your palate. Let your taste buds be your guide. The juice should taste robust and delicious.

- **Vegetable broth** is made from ripe, healthy vegetables and legumes simmered together in a pot for several hours. You may add sea salt, soy sauce (if tolerated), capers, and such spices as oregano, basil, thyme, or curry to suit your taste. The clear broth should be strained and may be drunk at any temperature. It will stay fresh for several days if refrigerated.

- **Water:** Drink deep springwater, naturally carbonated water, and water with citrus juice.

- **Herbal teas** are welcome additions to this program.

You will want to remain on a liquid-only diet for one to three days. You may want to start this plan on a long weekend or when you are on vacation, since you will need frequent access to a refrigerator and some kitchen equipment. In addition, by starting the program on a weekend, you can avoid any conflicts at work if you feel irritable or grouchy.

WHAT YOU NEED TO KNOW ABOUT FAT

No discussion of diet can escape a mention of dietary fat. While many diets focus on how much fat you should consume, the IBS Eating Plan focuses on the quality rather than the quantity of fat. As a general rule, you should avoid saturated fats and trans-fatty acids in favor of monounsaturated and polyunsaturated fats.

You must be on the lookout for trans fats, which are commonly used in processed foods. Food manufacturers hydrogenate the fats and oils they put into crackers and cakes and other foods so that they can start with cheap, low-quality oils and turn them into products that will not spoil on the grocery shelf. Trans fats have been shown to increase cholesterol, decrease beneficial high-density lipoprotein (HDL) cholesterol, interfere with the liver's detoxification system, and interfere with the function of the essential fatty acids. Any food that stresses the body in this way contributes to IBS by adding to the body's toxic load.

Some fats are, however, beneficial. Essential fatty acids, which are good for you, are abundant in plants and their seeds, including flaxseed, walnut, olive, sunflower, safflower, corn, canola, and evening primrose. They're also found in the fat of cold-water fish, including salmon, mackerel, sardines, tuna, and herring.

The most important essential fatty acids are the omega-3 and omega-6, which are named for their chemical configurations. Most people with fatty acid problems are deficient in omega-3 oils. The symptoms of such deficiency include cracking fingertips, dull patches of skin, mixed oily and dry skin, chicken skin (bumps on the back of the arms), alligator skin on the lower legs, dry hair, dandruff, hair loss, soft and brittle fingernails.

Know Your Fats

Saturated fats should be avoided as much as possible. These fats raise the level of cholesterol in the blood, and they tend to stimulate colon contractions.

- **Monounsaturated—recommended:** Olive oil, canola oil, peanut oil, avocados, olives, peanuts, peanut butter, cashews, almonds, and pecans.
- **Polyunsaturated—acceptable in limited quantities:** Safflower oil, sunflower oil, corn oil, soybean oil, cottonseed oil, sesame oil, mayonnaise, walnuts, and fish oils.
- **Saturated—avoid:** Butter, meat fat, lard (pork fat), hydrogenated fat, cream, cheese, whole milk, coconut oil, palm kernel oil, and palm oil.
- **Trans fats—avoid:** Hydrogenated fats and partially hydrogenated fats.

While this chapter provides information on what foods to eat, many of my patients ask for details about exactly how to put this program into practice. The following chapter will provide meal plans and some simple recipes to help you implement the IBS Eating Plan.

Chapter 8

Meal Plans and Recipes to Make Eating Right Easier

One of the biggest problems with sticking to a diet—any diet—is boredom. No matter how much you may love beet greens and baked chicken, the time may come that you long to savor a bite of a forbidden food during dinner.

Don't despair: You will be able to eat a variety of foods in the first phase of the IBS Eating Plan, and then gradually you will be able to build a more diversified diet, rich in healthy whole foods. As described in chapter 7, Phase 1 includes about two dozen core foods, chosen because they are more alkaline and less allergenic than other foods.

It can be difficult to give up favorite foods that aren't on the core list, even temporarily, but most of my patients are so thrilled with the results of the diet that they joyfully change their eating habits. More than a few patients report that they feel better than they have for years after going on the IBS Eating Plan, even after just a few days. You will need to change your diet—your IBS symptoms should provide clear evidence that your current eating habits don't agree with you—but if you stick to the plan, you will find that the benefits of good health will more than make up for any foods you must give up.

PREPARING YOUR KITCHEN

If you're used to using packaged mixes, prepared foods, and frozen meals, then you will have to make some adjustments to your cooking style when you implement the IBS Eating Plan. That being said, the only way you relieve your IBS symptoms and improve your overall health is to take responsibility for planning and preparing healthy meals.

Before starting the IBS Eating Plan, clean out your kitchen pantry, throwing away foods that no longer have a place in your diet (especially if you find these foods tempting). Throw away (or donate to charity) the following foods, which are often responsible for dietary downfalls:

- Breads, cakes, muffins, and other yeast-containing foods
- Dairy foods and other foods containing dairy products
- Corn syrup
- Sugar (granulated, powdered, white, brown)
- Soft drinks (with or without sugar)
- Processed foods
- All foods containing hydrogenated and partially hydrogenated fats, palm kernel oil, and coconut oil
- Foods containing food coloring and additives

If these foods aren't in your home, you will find it much easier to avoid them and make good food choices. You should then go shopping, using the foods on the core list for Phase 1 as a shopping list (see chapter 7).

Know Your Grains

You will want to become familiar with various alternative grains, such as amaranth, quinoa, and buckwheat, because they are less acidic than other grains and also less allergenic. These grains are available in most health food stores as well as a growing number of grocery stores. In most recipes, you can substitute one cooked grain for another—for example, you could substitute cooked quinoa for cooked brown rice.

- **Amaranth:** This gluten-free food resembles a grain, but it is actually a seed. It has a grainy, nutty flavor. The whole seeds can be cooked into hot cereal, or it is available ground into flour, which can be used as a substitute for white or wheat flour in baking. Buy the flour fresh and store it in the refrigerator to prevent it from becoming rancid.

- **Buckwheat:** Once again, this gluten-free product isn't a grain at all; it is a plant related to rhubarb. It can be used to make buckwheat pancakes, waffles, or breads, or it can be ground into flour. Buckwheat soba noodles (found in the Oriental section of the supermarket or health food store) provide an alternative to traditional pasta, but check the product labels carefully since some brands of soba noodles contain wheat flour as well.

- **Millet:** This is a grain the size of sesame seeds that is widely used in Asia and Africa. It is less allergenic than wheat and other grains. Millet meal or flour can be used in baking; puffed millet can be used as a breakfast cereal.

- **Quinoa:** This seed is related to beets, spinach, and chard. Quinoa flour, available in health food stores, can be used as a grain substitute in baked products. The seeds can be cooked similarly to rice, but you should take the time to thoroughly wash off their bitter outer coating. To do so, swish the seeds vigorously in water until the water runs clear without foaming. The quinoa can then be cooked for fifteen minutes, using two cups of water for every one cup of grain.

- **Teff:** This is a nongluten grain from Africa. Available as both whole seeds and flour, teff makes an excellent wheat alternative. Cooked teff absorbs more water than most grains; cook with four cups of water for every one cup of grain.

TIME-SAVING TIPS

- Prepare a large fresh salad every other day. Use greens, onions, pine nuts, and tofu cubes. Have some when you need a quick and easy meal or snack.
- Make pesto for use as a dip with raw veggies, or as a topping for steamed veggies.
- Keep fresh lemons and limes on hand for use as a vinegar substitute and to flavor drinking water.

PHASE 1 MEAL PLANS: NO RECIPES NECESSARY

During Phase 1 of the IBS Eating Plan, your diet will include whole foods with few ingredients so that you will be able to identify any potential allergens without being confused about which ingredients may be problematic. By limiting your diet to relatively few low-allergenic foods, you will give your digestive system a chance to stabilize and recover from IBS. Most people find that their IBS symptoms subside within days of beginning Phase 1.

You won't need to follow recipes at first, because you will want to keep the foods you eat simple—steamed or stir-fried fresh vegetables; broiled, baked, or poached meat, fowl, or fish. Don't hesitate to eat chicken and brown rice for breakfast or dine on oatmeal with peaches for dinner.

Breakfast

- Oatmeal with fruit
- Brown rice with fruit
- Leftovers from previous dinner
- Ginger tea

Lunch or Dinner

- Salad with cucumbers and bean sprouts
- Pork (baked, broiled, poached)
- Chicken or turkey (baked, broiled, poached)
- Fish (baked, broiled, poached)
- Vegetables (raw, steamed, or stir-fried: asparagus, eggplant, beet greens, red peppers, spinach, or string beans)
- Brown rice
- Ginger tea

Snacks

- Nuts (almonds, cashews, chestnuts)
- Seeds (pumpkin)
- Fruit (organic watermelon, fresh peaches, fresh apricots)

INTO THE KITCHEN: A RECIPE SAMPLER FOR PHASES 2 AND 3

You won't have to give up taste to enjoy good health on the IBS Eating Plan. During Phase 2 and Phase 3, you will be able to experiment with more interesting food combinations. The recipes in this chapter feature delicious home-cooked dishes made with nutritious, whole foods. They can be worked into the meal plan for Phase 2 or Phase 3, once the necessary ingredients have been tested for food sensitivity by introducing them one at a time.

Breakfast

- Apple Chutney with Brown Rice (page 103)
- Breakfast Broccoli with Rice (page 104)
- Breakfast Waldorf Salad (page 105)
- Rise 'n' Shine Hot Cereal with Fruit (page 113)

Lunch or Dinner

- Black-Eyed Peas, Greens, and Millet (page 104)
- Chilled Eggplant Salad (page 105)
- Cold Cucumber Soup (page 106)
- Garbanzo Spread (page 107)
- Gazpacho (page 108)
- Guacamole with Fresh Veggies (page 110)
- Millet with Artichoke Hearts and Vegetables (page 110)
- Minestrone (page 111)
- Ratatouille (page 112)
- String Beans Vinaigrette (page 114)

- Turkey and Vegetable Salad (page 114)
- Vegetable Salad Wraps (page 115)
- Vegetable Steam-Fry (page 116)

Snacks

- Fruit Salad (page 107)
- Cucumber Salad (page 107)
- Raw broccoli and cauliflower with Pesto (page 112)
- Cashews, chestnuts, or almonds, unsalted
- Fresh whole fruit: nectarine, raspberries, watermelon, tangerine, or pineapple
- Pumpkin seeds, unsalted

APPLE CHUTNEY WITH BROWN RICE

1½ pounds cooking apples
1 clove garlic, minced
1 tablespoon chopped gingerroot
½ cup fresh-squeezed orange juice
1 teaspoon cinnamon
1 teaspoon ground cloves
1 teaspoon sea salt
1 cup apple cider vinegar
1 cup brown rice, cooked

Chop the apples into bite-size pieces. (You don't need to peel them.) Combine all the other ingredients, including the rice, in a heavy saucepan. Bring to a boil, then simmer, uncovered, for 1 hour. Cool. This recipe makes about 1 quart; it can be stored in the refrigerator for 2 weeks. Serve over brown rice.

BLACK-EYED PEAS, GREENS, AND MILLET

Vegetable cooking spray
1 medium onion, sliced
2 cloves garlic, minced
2 cups vegetable broth
3 tablespoons apple cider vinegar
6 cups turnip greens, chopped
2 large tomatoes, in wedges
15 ounces black-eyed peas
1 cup millet
2 tablespoons cilantro, finely chopped
Sea salt to taste

Spray a large saucepan with cooking spray; heat over medium heat until hot. Sauté the onion and garlic until tender, about 5 minutes. Add the broth and vinegar; heat to a boil. Add the greens and tomatoes to the saucepan; reduce the heat and simmer, covered, until the greens are wilted, about 5 minutes.

Stir the black-eyed peas and millet into the saucepan; simmer, covered, until all the liquid is absorbed, about 25 minutes. Remove from the heat and let stand for 5 minutes. Stir in the cilantro and season to taste.

BREAKFAST BROCCOLI WITH RICE

2 cups chopped broccoli
½ cup chopped onion
½ teaspoon sea salt
2 tablespoons olive oil
¼ teaspoon basil
¼ teaspoon black pepper
1 cup brown rice, cooked

Sauté the broccoli, onion, and salt in the olive oil until the broccoli is bright green. Add the herbs. Mix with the cooked rice and serve.

BREAKFAST WALDORF SALAD

3 apples, cored and cut into bite-size chunks
Juice of 2 lemons
1 large orange, in sections
1 stalk celery, chopped
½ cup toasted cashews
2 tablespoons raisins

Dressing:
1 cup unsweetened yogurt
1 small avocado, mashed
½ teaspoon freshly grated lemon rind

Soak the apples in half the lemon juice. Combine the juice from the second lemon with the dressing ingredients in a blender and process until smooth. Toss the remaining ingredients with the dressing.

CHILLED EGGPLANT SALAD

2 small eggplants
2 medium tomatoes
1 cucumber
1 green pepper
1 red pepper
Chopped parsley

Marinade:
2 cloves garlic, crushed
Juice of 3 lemons
¼ cup olive oil
¼ cup safflower oil
½ teaspoon sea salt
1 teaspoon basil
Black pepper to taste

Cut the eggplants into ½-inch slices, peel, and lightly salt. Broil on an oiled tray until brown on both sides; the eggplant will be tender when touched with a fork. Chop it into bite-size pieces. Mix all the ingredients for the marinade and cover the eggplant with the marinade. Chill for 2 hours. Before serving, chop the other vegetables and parsley into small chunks and mix with the eggplant.

COLD CUCUMBER SOUP

4 cups peeled, seeded, chopped cucumber
2 cups water
1 cup plain yogurt
1 clove garlic, minced
2 fresh mint leaves
1 teaspoon sea salt
¼ teaspoon dill weed
1 teaspoon chives

Puree all the ingredients in a blender. Refrigerate and serve cold.

CUCUMBER SALAD

2 cups chopped cucumbers
1 tablespoon parsley, chopped
1 tablespoon lemon juice
1 tablespoon flaxseed or olive oil
¼ cup finely chopped peppermint

In a small bowl, mix all the ingredients. Chill for several hours. Toss again before serving.

FRUIT SALAD

Chopped watermelon
Raspberries
Grapes
Nectarines
Mangos
Papaya
Pears
Tangerines
Raspberries
Pineapple chunks

Combine the fruits in any proportions; do not include cranberries, plums, coconuts, or guavas. Chill for several hours.

GARBANZO SPREAD

2 cups canned garbanzo beans (chickpeas)
1 chopped medium onion

2 tablespoons dried parsley
1 teaspoon sea salt
1 teaspoon coriander
Dash of chili powder
¼ cup water

Blend all the ingredients in a blender until smooth. Spread on sprouted whole wheat tortillas and top with fresh vegetables.

GAZPACHO

4 cups tomato juice
1 minced onion
1 cucumber, diced
2 scallions, chopped
¼ cup chopped green bell pepper
¼ cup finely chopped celery
1 tablespoon olive oil
½ teaspoon pepper
1 teaspoon basil
1 clove garlic, minced
Juice of ½ lemon
Sea salt

Combine all the ingredients; cover and chill overnight. The soup can be pureed, if desired.

GHEE—"LIQUID GOLD"

1 pound unsalted butter

Ghee, or clarified butter, is often called liquid gold. It is excellent for cooking because it does not bubble or smoke, it contains no additives, yet it does not turn rancid. Since the whey is removed during preparation, it is acceptable for people with milk intolerance.

To make ghee, place a pound of good-quality (grade AA) unsalted butter in a heavy saucepan. Allow the butter to melt, either on top of the stove or in the oven. Stirring occasionally, bring the butter to a boil. When a layer of foam covers the surface, lower the heat and continue to cook undisturbed for about 1 hour on top of the stove or slightly longer (about 1½ hours) in the oven. By then the butter will have separated. Under the layer of solid white surface foam will be amber-colored clarified butter (ghee), and at the bottom of the saucepan will be some sediment. What has happened is the water has evaporated, and the protein solids have separated from the original butter.

Without shaking the saucepan, use a fine-mesh wire skimmer to carefully skim off as much foam as you can from the surface. Then strain the clear liquid ghee through several layers of cheesecloth to remove the remaining foam. Ladle the clarified ghee into a clean glass jar or crock with a tight-fitting lid. Refrigerate or freeze the ghee. At low temperature, the ghee will become solid. One pound of butter will yield about 1⅔ cups (¾ pound) of ghee.

Use ghee as you would butter or oil, for sautéing, braising, or in combination with cooked vegetables, legumes, and casseroles. Ghee can be heated to a higher temperature than most oils or fats without the problems of bubbling and smoking.

Ghee is superior to other animal and vegetable fats. Research has shown that ghee does not raise blood cholesterol levels. Ghee is also commercially available at health food stores.

GUACAMOLE WITH FRESH VEGGIES

2 ripe avocados, mashed
Juice of 1 lemon
2 cloves garlic, crushed
Minced green pepper
1 small finely minced onion
1 small chopped cucumber
½ teaspoon sea salt
Black pepper, to taste
Fresh seasonal veggies, for dipping

Mix all the ingredients (except the veggies) together and chill.

MILLET WITH ARTICHOKE HEARTS AND VEGETABLES

½ cup millet
1¾ cups vegetable broth, divided
2 cans artichoke hearts, drained and halved
1 tablespoon olive oil
¼ teaspoon garlic powder
2 medium onions, chopped
1 medium green bell pepper, chopped
2 cloves garlic, minced
2 medium tomatoes, chopped
1 medium eggplant, unpeeled, cut into 1-inch cubes
1 medium zucchini, sliced

2 tablespoons parsley, finely chopped
Sea salt to taste

Cook the millet in a large skillet over medium heat until toasted, 2 minutes. Add 1¼ cups of the broth and heat to a boil; reduce the heat and simmer, covered, until the millet is tender and the broth is absorbed, about 15 minutes. Remove from the heat and let stand, covered, for 10 minutes.

Sauté the artichokes in the olive oil in a large skillet until well browned on all sides, 5 minutes. Remove from the skillet and sprinkle with garlic powder.

Add the onions, green pepper, and garlic to the skillet. Sauté until tender, 3 to 5 minutes. Add the remaining ½ cup broth along with the remaining vegetables and parsley; heat to a boil. Reduce the heat and simmer, covered, until the eggplant is tender, 15 to 20 minutes.

Add the millet and artichoke hearts to the skillet; cook until hot through, 3 to 4 minutes. Season with salt.

MINESTRONE

1 cup chopped onion
3 cloves garlic, crushed
2 tablespoons olive oil
1 cup chopped celery
½ cup cubed carrots
1 cup cubed eggplant
1 teaspoon sea salt
1 teaspoon oregano
½ cup chopped fresh parsley, plus more for garnish
1 teaspoon basil
1 cup chopped green pepper
2 cups tomato puree

3½ cups water or vegetable stock
½ cup garbanzo beans
1 cup brown rice

In a soup kettle, sauté the onion and garlic in the olive oil until they are soft and translucent. Add the celery, carrots, eggplant, and salt. Mix well. Add the oregano, parsley, and basil. Cover and cook over low heat for 5 minutes. Add the green pepper, puree, stock, and beans. Cover and simmer for 15 minutes. Bring to a boil and add the rice, boiling until tender. Serve immediately, topped with extra parsley.

PESTO

6 cloves garlic
4 cups fresh basil or 1 cup dried basil
1 cup fresh parsley
6 tablespoons pine nuts
1 cup olive oil
½ teaspoon sea salt
½ teaspoon pepper
2 tablespoons sun-dried tomatoes

Combine all the ingredients in a food processor or blender. Blend until smooth.

RATATOUILLE

¼ cup olive oil
4 cloves garlic, crushed
1 medium onion, chopped
1 small eggplant, cubed

½ cup tomato juice
1 teaspoon basil
½ teaspoon oregano
2 small zucchini, cubed
2 medium bell peppers, in strips
2 teaspoons sea salt
2 medium tomatoes, chopped
2 tablespoons tomato paste
Fresh parsley, chopped, for garnish

Heat the olive oil in large cooking pot. Crush the garlic into the oil. Add the onion and sauté over medium heat until the onion turns transparent. Add the eggplant and tomato juice, then add the herbs. Stir to mix well, then cover and simmer for 10 to 15 minutes over low heat. When the eggplant is soft to the touch with a fork, add the zucchini and pepper. Cover and simmer for 10 minutes. Add the salt, tomatoes, and tomato paste. Mix well. Stew until all vegetables are tender. Garnish with fresh parsley before serving. This is excellent served over brown rice or another cooked grain of your choice.

RISE 'N' SHINE HOT CEREAL WITH FRUIT

1 cup quinoa
1 pear, chopped
1 apple, chopped
¼ cup chopped cashews
¼ teaspoon cinnamon
⅛ teaspoon ground cloves

Prepare the quinoa and mix with the chopped fruit, nuts, and spices. You can vary the recipe using different grains (millet, buckwheat, brown rice); different fruits (pineapple, berries, peaches, or any other fruit); and different types of nuts. This cereal can be prepared and divided into several morning meals; some people enjoy eating it cold as well. Be creative; this can be a staple of your morning meals.

STRING BEANS VINAIGRETTE

1 pound fresh green beans
½ medium onion
1 small clove garlic
6 tablespoons olive oil
2 tablespoons apple cider vinegar
½ teaspoon sea salt

Wash the beans, snip off the ends, and cut them French style. Drop them into boiling salted water and cook until just tender. Drain.

Finely chop the onion and mince the clove of garlic. Combine these with the beans and remaining ingredients and mix well. Chill and serve with tomatoes, olives, and other fresh or marinated garnishes of your choice.

TURKEY AND VEGETABLE SALAD

½ cup broccoli florets
2 tablespoons olive oil
1 tablespoon apple cider vinegar
¼ cup diced carrots
¼ cup diced zucchini
1 cup diced cooked turkey
1 cup brown rice, cooked
Sea salt and pepper to taste

Steam the broccoli for 5 minutes; rinse in cold water. Mix together the olive oil and vinegar. Add the vegetables, turkey, and rice. Season with salt and pepper, as desired.

VEGETABLE SALAD WRAPS

1¼ cups millet
3½ cups water
½ cup sliced celery
½ medium red bell pepper, sliced
4 green onions, sliced
1 medium carrot, sliced
¼ cup parsley, finely chopped
2 tablespoons fresh basil, chopped
1 medium tomato, chopped
½ head green leaf lettuce, sliced
1 head iceberg lettuce

Oregano Dressing:
3 tablespoons olive oil
3 tablespoons apple cider vinegar
1 teaspoon oregano

Cook the millet in a large saucepan over medium heat until toasted, 2 to 3 minutes. Add the water and heat to a boil; reduce the heat and simmer, covered, until the millet is tender and the liquid is absorbed, about 15 minutes. Remove from the heat and let stand, covered, for 10 minutes. Cool.

Combine the celery, bell pepper, green onions, carrot, parsley, and basil in a food processor; process, using the pulse technique, until finely chopped. Transfer to a large bowl.

Add the tomato and millet to the vegetable mixture and toss. Drizzle with Oregano Dressing and toss.

Wash the lettuce and separate into whole leaves. Place some of the vegetable mixture in the middle of each lettuce leaf and wrap as if you were preparing a burrito or sandwich wrap.

VEGETABLE STEAM-FRY

1 teaspoon grated fresh ginger
2 cloves garlic, crushed
½ cup chopped broccoli
½ cup sliced cauliflower
½ cup red pepper strips
½ cup sliced onion
½ cup chopped yellow squash
1 cup pea pods
1 cup fried tofu
¼ teaspoon sea salt

Sauce:
⅓ cup water or vegetable stock
1 teaspoon dried ginger
Juice of ½ lemon

Heat an electric frying pan. Add a small amount of water and steam-fry the ginger and garlic for a couple of minutes. Add the veggies, tofu, and salt and steam-fry until the veggies are bright and slightly softened. Pour the steam-fry sauce mixture over the top and steam for 1 minute more.

Chapter 9

Relax Your Mind, Relax Your Colon

By the time they come to me, most of my patients have spent years going from one doctor to another seeking help for their IBS. They have undergone dozens of tests and medical procedures, with inconclusive results. They have tried various prescription medications to alter the chemistry in their digestive system, but their symptoms repeatedly return. They tell me horror stories of how their doctors dismiss them with condescending remarks to the effect of "It's all in your head."

In truth, IBS is caused by food sensitivities and other dietary factors, although stress and emotional issues may also play a role. Dozens of studies have looked at the cause of IBS; most have concluded that the condition is a functional disorder aggravated by stress. In addition, IBS has been linked to anxiety disorders triggered by stress. Researchers at the Medical University of South Carolina reported in *The Journal of Clinical Psychiatry* (2001) that of people who seek treatment for IBS, 50 to 90 percent have psychiatric problems, including panic disorder, anxiety disorder, social phobia, depression, and post-traumatic stress disorder. In my experience, people can benefit from following the IBS Program outlined in this book, regardless of their psychiatric history.

Fortunately, you can do a great deal to minimize stress and to control your body's response to it. This chapter reviews the physiology of stress—what happens to your gastrointestinal tract and other body systems when you feel pressured and panicked—and it offers suggestions on techniques you can use to defuse the stress response.

HOW YOUR BODY REACTS TO STRESS

Life is stressful. To your body, stress is any challenge or change you confront. An auto accident is stressful, and so is buying a new car. Losing an important contest or missing out on a promotion is stressful, and so is winning or getting a promotion, no matter how well deserved. A divorce is stressful, and so is falling in love. And as people with IBS are well aware, living with a digestive problem is stressful in a number of ways. While you may not be able to avoid stress, you can control the way you respond to it so that it will no longer take an undue toll on your physical and psychological well-being.

Our understanding of how the body reacts to stress can be traced back to Walter B. Cannon, a physiologist at Harvard University at the turn of the twentieth century. Cannon first recognized and defined the so-called fight-or-flight response to stress, which involves a number of biochemical changes that happen to the body in preparation for dealing with danger. This response made sense in evolutionary terms: Early humans needed quick bursts of energy to escape danger or fight off life-threatening predators. Though modern people face fewer of these life-or-death threats, our bodies still respond to stressful events in much the same way as our prehistoric relatives.

In the body, any stressor (either real or imagined) causes the cerebral cortex of the brain to trigger an alarm to the hypothalamus in the midbrain. The hypothalamus then charges into action, sending messages throughout the body to prepare for an emergency. As a result, your heart rate increases, your breathing grows faster, your muscles tense, your metabolism kicks into high gear, and your blood pressure soars. Your hearing becomes more acute and your pupils dilate. Your digestive system also responds: Your mouth becomes dry, your stomach churns, or you feel the sudden need to clear your bowels. You're ready to deal with anything.

During this stress response, your body also releases adrenaline, epinephrine, cortisol, and other chemicals that prepare for danger, but also inhibit the immune system and interfere with digestion, reproduction, growth, and tissue repair. Prolonged or chronic stress creates a cascade of physiological responses that can ultimately result in IBS. Ongoing stress leads to adrenal fatigue, and the body becomes unable to make more of these hormones. This, in turn, causes a drop in levels of secretory IgA, antibodies that help keep the mucous membranes protected. This leads to leaky gut syndrome and leaves the body more vulnerable to developing food and chemical hypersensitivities, which in turn contributes to IBS.

In addition, the high level of adrenaline speeds up the metabolism of proteins, fats, and carbohydrates so that the body has plenty of energy to use during the emergency. To achieve this surge in energy, the body excretes amino acids, potassium, and phosphorus, draws magnesium from the muscle tissues, and fails to store needed calcium. Not surprisingly, during periods of stress, the body often becomes deficient in many key nutrients.

Prolonged stress also changes the chemistry of the digestive tract. At first, stress increases the production of hydrochloric acid in the stomach, causing indigestion, heartburn, gastritis, and ulcers. The pancreas, however, responds by releasing alkaline enzymes to help balance the acidity. With chronic stress, this can lead to hypochlorhydria (low stomach acid) and reduced function on the pancreas. Low stomach acid results in poor digestion and assimilation of nutrients, which can contribute to the development of leaky gut syndrome and food allergies (as discussed in chapter 4).

At the same time that stress is changing the acid content of the stomach, it is also disrupting the acid–alkaline balance in the body. When oxygen is diverted from the stomach to the other organs during times of stress, the stomach cannot produce enough digestive enzymes to thoroughly digest food and dispose of metabolic wastes. This excessively acidic waste moves into the intestines, which lack the thick mucous lining found in the stomach. (The lining of the intestines is designed to be thinner so that it can allow digested food to pass through the intestinal walls to the blood and lymphatic systems.) This acidic waste inflames the intestinal lining and kills the friendly bacteria necessary for microbial harmony. When the harmful bacteria take over, they further damage the intestinal lining by releasing poisonous wastes that include alcohol, ammonia, acetaldehyde, and formaldehyde.

Fortunately, it is relatively easy for the body to flip a switch and reverse the stress response. Your body begins to relax as soon as your brain receives the signal that the danger has passed and it's safe to relax. The brain cancels the emergency signals to the central nervous system, and within about three minutes the panic messages cease and relaxation begins. The heart rate and breathing slow, and the other systems return to their normal levels.

Your body can't tell whether the relaxation response was triggered by a change in circumstances or a change in your attitude. Either way, the relaxation is the same. Just as chronic, prolonged stress can make IBS symptoms more intense, so reversing stress can help promote relaxation and relax the bowel.

As part of learning to control your IBS, you can learn techniques for reducing anxiety by taking time for mental calming and the release of daily stress. The self-help techniques on page 122 can be very helpful in promoting relaxation.

TYPES OF STRESS

- **Physical stress:** Exercise, physical labor, childbirth.

- **Environmental stress:** Exposure to pollutants, pesticides, chemicals, drugs, alcohol, caffeine, nicotine.

- **Mental stress:** Anxiety, worry, long work hours, lack of control, perfectionism, mental illness.

- **Emotional stress:** Anger, fear, frustration, grief, betrayal.

- **Nutritional stress:** Vitamin and mineral deficiencies, food allergies, overeating.

- **Traumatic stress:** Illness, infection, injury, surgery.

- **Psychological stress:** Relationship problems, financial pressures, job challenges, overall outlook on life.

OKAY, RELAX

Some relaxation techniques can be practiced at home with little instruction; others require assistance, training, or special equipment. The suggestions made in this chapter can help you manage stress and minimize stress-related IBS.

Techniques You Can Try on Your Own

Breathing

Most people take their breathing for granted. But breathing is actually a complex process involving the transfer of oxygen to the tissues and the removal of the waste product carbon dioxide. Deep breathing helps relax the body and quiet the mind.

When people are under stress, they often breathe poorly, taking shallow, weak breaths. With an inadequate supply of oxygen (and the inadequate removal of waste products), the body is less able to manage stress, resulting in anxiety, panic attacks, depression, headaches, fatigue, and muscle tension. On the other hand, healthful deep breathing helps relax the body and quiet the mind. Good breathing techniques can be practiced separately or along with other relaxation exercises.

Consider what happens inside your body when you draw a breath: The air is pulled in through your nose, where the nasal passages warm it to body temperature, filter out foreign particles, and add a touch of humidity to keep the lungs moist. In the lungs, the air travels along a series of tubes or branches to tiny air sacs called alveoli, which inflate when air fills the lungs and contract when air is exhaled. Blood vessels and capillaries next to the alveoli absorb the oxygen and pass it on to the heart. In the heart, the oxygenated blood is pumped out and distributed throughout the body. The blood cells then trade fresh oxygen for carbon dioxide, which returns to the heart and works its way back through the capillaries to the alveoli, through the lungs, and out of the body as you exhale.

When people are nervous or stressed, they usually engage in chest breathing, which tends to be shallow, rapid, and irregular, involving only the top part of the lungs. When a chest breather draws in the air, the chest expands and the shoulders rise, but the air does not entirely fill the lungs. This results in inadequate oxygenation of the blood, which causes the heart rate to increase and stress to build.

Abdominal breathing is the natural pattern for newborn babies and sleeping adults, but most adults don't do it during their waking hours. To properly nourish and oxygenate the lungs, air should be drawn deeply into the lungs, allowing the chest to fill entirely with air and the belly to rise and fall slowly. Breathing should be even and unrestricted.

When you become aware of your breathing, you will inhale more fully and feel the muscle tension and stress melt away. You will experience a greater sense of calm and well-being almost immediately as you feel the improved oxygenation in your tissues.

Go ahead and take a deep breath. Fill your lungs with air, then slowly exhale. Do it again. Put one hand on your abdomen and the other on the center of your chest. Without attempting to change your breathing pattern, take note of how you are breathing. Then move on to concentrated, deep abdominal breathing.

Whenever you practice deep breathing, if you experience

shortness of breath, heart palpitations, or a feeling that you can't get enough air, stop immediately and return to your regular breathing pattern.

Meditation

Meditation comes in a variety of forms and traditions, but at the most basic level the practice involves attempting to focus your complete attention on one thing at a time. As most people discover when they try meditation, the mind tends to wander; it can be challenging to remain focused on a single object without distracting thoughts interfering with the concentration.

This back-and-forth struggle for control of the thoughts is not only natural, but can also be therapeutic: It teaches the person meditating that there is a choice about what to think about and how to feel. Eventually it becomes clear that it is impossible to feel tense or angry or hostile when your mind is focused somewhere else. Meditation helps you relax because your mind no longer dwells on the negative stimulus since it is busy thinking about the target object.

Research has shown that meditation helps the body relax. For example, back in 1968 researchers at Harvard Medical School found that when people practiced Transcendental Meditation (a type of mantra meditation), their heart rate and breathing slowed, their oxygen consumption dropped by 20 percent, their blood lactate levels dropped, their skin resistance to electrical current increased, and their brain wave patterns showed greater alpha wave activity—all physiological signs of deep relaxation.

To experiment with the technique of meditation, find a

quiet place where you are not apt to be interrupted. Sit in a firm chair with your back as straight as possible. (You may prefer lying down flat on the ground, depending on the type of meditation you will be doing.)

There are three common forms of meditation, each with a different object of focus:

- **Mantra meditation** involves repeating (either aloud or silently) a word, syllable, or group of words. Each time you breathe out, you recite a neutral syllable (such as *ommm*) or a soothing word (such as *peace* or *calm*) or a phrase (such as *it's okay*).

- **Gazing meditation** involves looking at an object such as a candle flame, a stone, or a flower to keep your attention focused. The object should be about one foot away from your face. Gaze at it rather than stare, keeping your eyes relaxed. Don't try to think about the object in words; just look at it without judgment.

- **Breathing meditation** involves focusing on the rising and falling of your breath. Some people consider this the most relaxing form of meditation. Draw a deep breath, focusing on the inhalation, the pause before your exhale, the exhalation, and the pause before your inhale again. When you exhale, say to yourself, "One." Each time you complete a breath and exhale, count again, one through four, then start over with one. The counting helps clear your mind of other thoughts.

With each type of meditation, start the session by inhaling deeply and pausing to enjoy the feeling of fullness. Then exhale fully, imagining that you are releasing all the tension in your body. During the time of meditation, if thoughts about your daily life slip into your mind (and they will when you are first starting out), accept them and let them drift away without worry.

Try meditating for five to ten minutes at first, then work up to fifteen to twenty minutes once or twice a day. The more you practice, the better you'll get at freeing your mind of cluttering thought. At the end of the session, you should feel much more relaxed and calm.

For more information about meditation, refer to books in the library or contact:

Cambridge Insight Meditation Center
331 Broadway
Cambridge, MA 02139
(617) 491-5070
www.cimc.info

Foundation of Human Understanding
P.O. Box 1009
Grants Pass, OR 97526
(800) 866-8883; (503) 597-4360
www.fhu.com

The Mind/Body Medical Institute
824 Boylston Street
Chestnut Hills, MA 02467
(617) 991-0102
www.mbni.org

The Foundation for Human Understanding
P.O. Box 1009
Grants Pass, OR 97526
(503) 597-4360
www.fhu.com

Progressive Relaxation

Done properly, progressive relaxation can lead to profound calm. Start by lying on your back on the floor, with your legs flat and your arms loose at your sides. Close your eyes and breathe deeply.

Once you are calm, you can begin systematically to tense and relax every muscle in your body. Start with your feet; tense the muscles in your feet for thirty seconds or so, then relax, allowing your feet to feel heavy and relaxed. Then move on to your calves, thighs, abdomen, buttocks, hands, forearms, upper arms, shoulders, and face.

When you finish, your muscles should feel soothed and relaxed. Lie quietly and enjoy the feeling of complete relaxation.

This technique is helpful because most people do not realize which of their muscles are chronically tense. By working through the muscles in the body, the technique helps people identify particular muscles and muscle groups that tend to collect tension and stress.

Visualization

You can reduce stress with a tremendously powerful tool you always have at your disposal: your imagination. Through visualization, you can ease the symptoms of stress by changing your thoughts. This practice builds on the idea that you are what you think you are. All your thoughts become reality. For example, if you think anxious thoughts, you become tense; if you think sad thoughts, you become unhappy. On the other hand, if you think soothing, positive thoughts, you will feel relaxed and have a more positive outlook.

Visualization can bring on a deep state of relaxation if you're willing and able to use your imagination creatively. Sit down in a comfortable position or lie on the floor in a quiet, dimly lit room. Tense all your muscles at once and hold for thirty seconds. Remember to breathe deeply as you contract your muscles. Then relax every muscle and allow all the tension to drain from your body. Continue to inhale and exhale slowly and fully.

Now that you have relaxed your muscles, you can begin the visualization part of the exercise. First, concentrate on your breathing, feeling the regular rhythm of each breath. Clear your mind of all thoughts, then imagine that you are in a peaceful setting—walking along a sandy beach, lying in a meadow of wildflowers on a spring day, or looking out over an evergreen mountain range. Use all your senses: Smell the ocean mist, feel the warm sun caress your back. The more specific your fantasy, the more real it will seem. And the more real it seems, the more likely the tension will melt away.

At the end of the session, which should last about twenty minutes, gradually bring yourself back to "real time." When you open your eyes and get back to your daily routine, you will probably feel at ease, relaxed, and refreshed.

Techniques You Can Try with Assistance

Biofeedback

Biofeedback involves training yourself to use your mind to voluntarily control the body's internal systems. The key to biofeedback is practice, so that you can learn the precise effect of mind over body. To learn the skill, you attach electrodes to various parts of your body to measure your heart rate, blood pressure, temperature, muscle tension, and brain wave patterns. A small machine on the other end of the wires displays the data, usually in the form of pictures, graphic lines, or audible beeps. You can literally watch yourself relax or grow tenser.

To learn to relax, patients learn to produce alpha brain wave patterns. In this case the electrodes attach to an electroencephalograph, which displays the brain waves on an oscilloscope. When alpha waves are present, the machine sounds a tone. The patient's quest is to sustain the tone by holding on to the thought or visualization that proves soothing and relaxing. Most people can learn to produce alpha brain waves in a few training sessions with a biofeedback clinician.

By carefully studying the measurable changes in your body as you relax and change your thoughts, you can actually learn to slow yourself down and control your body's internal processes. This training in mind over matter can be very useful in learning to relax. Most of us have no trouble learning how to be stressed out, but it takes hours of practice to learn to slow down physiologically.

The goal, of course, is to become so familiar with the sensations associated with a particular physical state that you can control your body without being hooked up to the machine. Biofeedback can be quite successful in the treatment of IBS. Researchers at the Royal Free Hospital in London in 1998 used a biofeedback computer game designed to teach deep relaxation to people with severe IBS. The forty people in the study experienced marked improvement of their IBS symptoms after four thirty-minute sessions.

If you'd like to try biofeedback, ask your physician for a referral to an outpatient clinic or consult the organization listed below. Before making an appointment, ask about fees and whether or not the service would be covered by your health insurance plan.

For a referral to someone with expertise in biofeedback, contact:

The Association for Applied Psychophysiology and Biofeedback
10200 West 44th Avenue, Suite 304
Wheat Ridge, CO 80033
(303) 422-8436
www.aapb.org

Hypnosis

Hypnosis can be used to help you relax and control your response to stress. You can learn to build a relaxation response so that you can stop the physical symptoms of stress and overcome the digestive responses before they escalate into a full-blown IBS episode. In 2002, researchers at the University of North Carolina found that hypnosis can be quite effective in treating IBS symptoms.

First, get over the horror-movie image of the evil hypnotist putting the unwitting patient into a sleepy-eyed trance. In truth, during hypnosis the participant is in a highly alert state, deeply concentrating on the suggestions of the hypnotist. In most hypnosis sessions, you would start by closing your eyes and thinking relaxing thoughts. The hypnotist would then guide you into deeper states of relaxation and focused concentration.

At this point, you are well aware of everything going on around you, but you are also more open to the power of suggestion. In such a state, you may be more responsive to suggestions of new ways to calm your bowels when you first feel them start to rumble.

Of course, hypnosis doesn't always work; some people are more responsive to the approach than others. But it is estimated that at least half of the people who try hypnosis respond after several sessions.

If you want to try stress management through hypnosis, ask your doctor for a referral to a psychiatrist or therapist qualified in the field. Don't just look in the phone book; many states have no licensing requirements for hypnotists. If your doctor can't make a referral, consider contacting one or more of the following professional organizations:

American Board of Hypnotherapy
2002 East McFadden Avenue, Suite 100
Santa Ana, CA 92705
(800) 872-9996; (714) 245-9340
www.hypnosis.com

American Council of Hypnotist Examiners
1147 East Broadway, Suite 340
Glendale, CA 91205
(818) 242-1159
www.hypnosisonline.com

American Society of Clinical Hypnosis
140 North Bloomingdale Road
Bloomingdale, IL 60108
(630) 980-4740
www.asch.com

National Guild of Hypnotists
P.O. Box 308
Merrimack, NH 03054-0308
(603) 429-9438
www.ngh.net

Massage

Massage can be a very effective way of reducing stress. The technique, which involves soothing touch of the muscles, soft tissues, and ligaments of the body, helps stimulate blood circulation and lower blood pressure.

There are two main types of massage: shiatsu and Swedish. Shiatsu involves finger massage at key points of the body, very much like acupressure. The technique was developed in Japan at roughly the same time as acupressure was being refined in China.

Swedish massage includes four distinctive types of movements, each including continual, rhythmic motions and constant contact with the body. The techniques include:

- **Effleurage:** This touch involves rhythmic, soothing strokes with open hands, the heels and palms, or the thumbs. In some cases, massage oil or cream is used to make motions smooth and even.

- **Percussion:** This technique includes brisk motions with alternate hands, such as chopping, pummeling, clapping, or tapping. It stimulates the skin and promotes circulation.

- **Petrissage:** This type of touch includes kneading, rolling, squeezing, lifting, and pressing the skin to stretch and stimulate the muscles. One hand should release its grip when the other takes over.

- **Pressure:** This technique involves focused pressure, using small circular movements made with the thumbs, fingertips, or heel of the hand. It should be used at local tension spots or knotted muscles. The pressure should be held for about ten seconds, followed by effleurage to soothe the area.

You can learn massage techniques yourself, either by checking out a book from the library or by taking a class. You might also consider consulting a massage therapist, who should know a variety of techniques. Most states require licensing of massage therapists; if your state doesn't, look for a therapist with certification from a professional organization. For information on state licensing requirements and a list of certified massage therapists in your area, call the National Certification Board for Therapeutic Massage and Board for Therapeutic Massage and Bodywork at (800) 296-0664. You can also contact:

American Massage Therapy Association
820 Davis Street, Suite 100
Evanston, IL 60201
(708) 864-0123
www.amtamassage.org

American Oriental Bodywork Therapy Association
1010 Haddonfield-Berlin, Suite 408
Voorhees, NY 08043
(856) 782-1616
www.aobta.org

Associated Bodywork and Massage Professionals
1271 Sugarbush Drive
Evergreen, CO 80439-9766
(800) 458-2267; (303) 674-8478
www.abmp.com

Yoga

Yoga promotes relaxation while at the same time strengthening and stretching the muscles. This form of exercise combines deep breathing with systematically moving the body into a series of postures, or positions. It can be very gentle and noncompetitive, making it an ideal exercise for people who may have grown out of shape over the years.

But yoga isn't easy. It requires significant endurance, strength, and flexibility. Since it works every muscle group, weaknesses can be identified easily, allowing you to target problem areas that may need special attention.

Another good option is Gi Gong (also known as Qi

Gong), the study and development of the body's natural energy to improve mental and physical health through the practice of specific breathing techniques. Breathing is used to open up the acupuncture meridians, allowing energy to flow to all parts of the body.

For background on yoga postures and Gi Gong, consider taking a class at a local recreation facility. You may also want to check out a videotape from your local library. Or contact:

Integral Yoga Institute
227 West 13th Street
New York, NY 10011
(212) 929-0586
www.integralyogany.org

Regular exercise can also help relieve stress and symptoms of IBS. The following chapter describes the benefits of exercise and offers advice on starting an exercise program that will both strengthen your digestive system and improve your overall health.

Chapter 10

Exercise for a Healthy Body and Healthy Bowel

You already know that exercise is good for you. You know that it's good for your heart and lungs, it strengthens and tones your muscles, and it helps prevent disease. But here's another reason to get off the couch and get moving: Regular exercise can relieve your IBS symptoms and improve your digestive health. In fact, just half an hour of moderate exercise such as aerobic walking four or five times a week may be all it takes to make you feel better.

Time and again I have seen how exercise helps relieve IBS symptoms among my patients. Regular exercise helps promote normal intestinal function, which in turn helps with the passage of gas, reduces bloating and cramping, and results in more regular bowel habits. A study published in the May 2001 issue of the journal *Gastroenterology Nursing* found that women with IBS were significantly less likely to be active than women in a control group.

THE MANY BENEFITS OF EXERCISE

Most of my patients—even those who hate to break a sweat—say they will start exercising if it will help ease their IBS symptoms. Of course, there are many other reasons to start working out. Exercise can improve your physical and emotional health, reduce your risk of serious illness, and make you look years younger than your chronological age. Studies have shown that moderate exercise strengthens the body's defenses against disease; after a workout, the number and aggressiveness of the white blood cells increase by 50 to 300 percent. In addition, exercise can:

- Reduce your risk of developing certain cancers, cardiovascular disease, colds and upper respiratory tract infections, diabetes (non-insulin-dependent), high blood pressure, obesity, osteoarthritis, osteoporosis, and stroke.
- Relieve anxiety, constipation, depression, low-back pain, and stress.
- Improve your cholesterol levels; lymphatic flow; flexibility; immune system; mental alertness and reaction time; mood; muscle strength; self-esteem; sexual desire, performance, and satisfaction; short-term memory; sleep; state of relaxation; vision; and overall quality of life.

You don't have to spend hours in the gym to enjoy these benefits. Recent studies have shown that as little as thirty minutes a day of light physical activity will reduce your risk of disease by lowering blood pressure and cholesterol. Yes, that's physical activity, not hard-core exercise. The time you spend strolling the neighborhood, walking the dog, climbing the stairs, and mowing the lawn counts toward your goal. Other studies have shown that you don't even have to do your thirty minutes of activity all at once.

Of course, these studies looked at minimum levels of exercise. To enjoy all the benefits of exercise, you'll have to work harder and longer. But the point is that with a nominal level of exertion, you can enjoy major lifesaving improvements in your overall health.

A FEW GOOD INTESTINAL EXERCISES

While regular workouts need to be part of an overall exercise plan, the following simple exercises can help relieve your IBS symptoms when your digestion is off. They can be used in addition to an overall exercise program, described later in this chapter.

- **Stomach flapping:** Stand up with your hands on your knees. Lean over slightly. Inhale. Exhale fully. With your breath held out, pull your stomach in as far as it will go, then suddenly release it all the way out—"flap it out." Repeat this flapping ten times on one exhalation. Repeat three times.

- **Abdominal roll:** Stand up. Roll your abdomen and pelvis around in circles, first to the right, then to the left. Do ten circles to the right, then ten circles to the left. While you are moving, with lightly closed fists gently drum, or lightly tap, your abdomen.

- **Intestinal hand massage:** Lie down and relax. Think of your favorite place. Pretend you are there. With the three middle fingers of each hand, gently massage your abdomen in little circles. Massage up your right side, across the top beneath your ribs, and down the left side to your pubic bone. If you feel any tension, tightness, or pain, work it out (gently rubbing until you feel the tension relax). Take a moment to inhale into the area and imagine that your healthy breath is relaxing the area.

- **Child's pose:** Sit on your heels with your knees spread slightly and lean forward until your forehead touches the floor. Relax like this for several minutes. Put your arms by your side. Gently inhale and exhale. This simple position gently stimulates and relaxes your intestinal tract. This is good for constipation.

- **Abdominal windmill:** Lie on your back. Bring your knees up to your chest. Place both knees to your right, touching the floor on your right side. Then, keeping your knees together, revolve to the left, touching the floor on your left side. If you need to, hold your knees together with your hands, and if you need to help move your knees with your hands, do so. Repeat ten to twenty times. Relax.

- **Cobra pose:** Lie on the floor on your stomach with your hands by your armpits and your elbows up toward the ceiling. Slowly push your palms against the floor, and lift your head and shoulders forward and upward. Lift yourself up as high as you can, while keeping your stomach and waist on the floor. Do not strain. Push your palms against the floor and try to create the sensation that you are stretching your abdomen in the direction you are facing, lengthening it out away from your waist. This is a healthy stretch for the abdominal area and enhances circulation and healing of this area.

DESIGNING AN OVERALL WORKOUT

A well-rounded exercise program strives to build aerobic fitness, muscle strength, and flexibility. While you won't necessarily do all types of exercise during every workout, your weekly routine should include all three types of exercise. You should wait two to two and a half hours after eating to exercise to minimize the impact of exercise on digestion.

Aerobic Fitness

If you don't exercise regularly, you have almost certainly lost aerobic power—and you probably know it. Without exercise, you will steadily lose aerobic conditioning throughout your thirties, forties, and fifties. By age sixty-five, the average person's aerobic capacity has dropped by about 40 percent compared to the relatively fit days of young adulthood. Climbing a flight of stairs or walking through an airport concourse—activity that once caused little exertion—might now leave you winded and strained.

The term *aerobic* means "using oxygen." During aerobic exercise, your heart and lungs work harder than normal to provide your muscles with the oxygen they demand, and you must breathe heavily and steadily to meet your body's increased need for oxygen. During anaerobic exercise, your heart and lungs cannot meet your body's oxygen demands for longer than a short burst of activity, and you are left gasping and wheezing for breath (even if you're in good shape). Jogging around a track is aerobic exercise; sprinting to catch the bus is anaerobic exercise. No one can do anaerobic exercise for more than a couple of minutes.

To improve your levels of aerobic fitness and strengthen your heart and lungs, you need to perform some type of aerobic exercise, such as walking, jogging, bicycling, swimming, cross-country skiing, aerobic dancing, or rope skipping. These activities involve the rhythmic, repeated use of the major muscle groups. When done regularly—three times a week for at least twenty to thirty minutes—aerobic activities improve the efficiency of the heart, lungs, and muscles and increase their ability to do work and withstand stress.

Walking, jogging, swimming laps, bicycling or riding an exercise bike, cross-country skiing (on skis or a skiing machine), rowing, in-line skating, aerobic dance, water aerobics, jumping rope, and stair climbing (either on a stair-step machine or on real stairs) are all good examples of aerobic activities. Tennis, soccer, racquetball, volleyball, basketball, golfing, ballroom dancing, gardening, lawn mowing, raking leaves, washing and waxing your car, or pushing a stroller can be used to supplement your aerobic exercise regimen.

Regular aerobic exercise helps lower your pulse rate, both during exercise and at rest. As your heart grows larger and stronger, it pumps more blood with each beat, decreasing blood pressure. One study found that older people who had already suffered a heart attack reduced their risk of a second attack by 20 to 25 percent when they started to exercise. These heart-saving benefits show up after as little as six to ten weeks of regular aerobic exercise.

For maximum benefit, you need to work hard enough—but not too hard. Your pulse rate, or the number of heartbeats per minute, is your body's speedometer: It tells you how fast your heart is going and if you need to speed up or slow things down to exercise in your optimal conditioning zone. Cardiovascular conditioning takes place when your heart beats at 70 to 85 percent of its maximum safe rate. Your maximum heart rate is approximately 220 minus your age. (See the table below.) You should take your pulse before starting to exercise, again after exercising for ten or fifteen minutes, and immediately after stopping.

Ideally, measure your heart rate with a heart monitor using a belt around the waist. If this is not available, you can measure your heart rate at any place where you can feel your pulse. Two easy pulse points are the inside wrist and the carotid artery in the neck. Using a stopwatch, count your pulse for ten seconds, then multiply this number by six to get the number of beats per minute. During exercise, a pulse that is under your target range indicates you should speed up or work harder, while one that is higher means you should slow down. Another simple test: You should be able to talk comfortably during exercise; if you can't carry on a conversation, you're working too hard.

Target Pulse Ranges

Age	Maximum Heart Rate	Target Range
40	180	126–153
45	175	122–140
50	170	119–145
55	165	115–140
60	160	112–136
65	155	109–132
70	150	105–128
75	145	102–123
80	140	98–119

If you're new to exercise, start slow. Try ten minutes of light to moderate exercise three times a week and gradually extend your workout time to twenty or thirty minutes, then increase intensity.

Aim for workouts of moderate intensity—about 70 percent of your maximum heart rate. If you work at the higher end of the exercise benefit zone, you will experience a faster improvement in your athletic ability, but this extra effort won't markedly improve your health, and it greatly increases your risk of injury. Moderate exercise reduces stress, anxiety, and blood pressure as effectively as strenuous exercise does.

Be sure to warm up for ten minutes by doing light calisthenics before your aerobic workout. You might also go through the motions of the main workout at a slower pace as a warm-up.

Also remember to cool down. After your workout, walk slowly for five to ten minutes, or until your heart rate returns to just ten to fifteen beats above its resting rate. (The more fit you are, the faster your heart rate will return to normal.) Stopping suddenly can cause the blood to pool in the legs, reducing blood pressure and possibly causing fainting or even a heart attack.

One word of caution: If you have heartburn, be aware that the kinds of exercise in which you jump up and down or bounce a lot—such as jogging, aerobic dancing, or using a stair-stepping machine—will stimulate your condition. I recommend to patients who have heartburn that they try nonjarring types of low-impact exercise, such as swimming or walking, to encourage healthy bowel motility and relieve stress and anxiety.

Get Walking

I recommend brisk walking for at least thirty minutes three or four times a week as one of the best forms of exercise. It's easy: Other than good shoes, you don't need special equipment, clothing, or facilities. You can walk almost anywhere in almost any weather, if you dress properly. Keep these tips in mind:

- Always walk facing traffic.
- Walk on sidewalks where possible, or stay close to the side of the road.
- Wear reflective clothing and carry a flashlight if you're walking after dark.
- Carry identification, but leave expensive jewelry and watches at home.
- Walk with a companion whenever possible, especially in a deserted area.
- If you walk alone, let someone know you're going walking, your routine, and when you expect to return.
- Don't use headphones if you're walking alone in an unfamiliar area, exercising at night, or in heavy traffic.
- Apply sunscreen if you'll be walking during the day to avoid sunburn.

Cleansing the Lymphatic System

Another benefit to exercise is its positive effect on the lymphatic system. Exercise effectively pumps the lymph through the body, moving toxins through the lymphatic system and releasing them from the body. This detoxification process helps relieve the symptoms of IBS by easing the toxic burden on the digestive system as well as the rest of the body.

The lymph has two big jobs in the human body. First, it delivers the immune cells to their sites of activity. Second, it eliminates toxins from the system—minimizing pathogens, by-products of metabolism, and any kind of pollution that's gotten into the interior of the system. The lymphatic system filters toxins out of the body, rather than allowing them to linger in the waste channels.

When you exercise and breathe deeply, you are pumping the lymph, the fluid that eliminates waste and activates immunity. Movement does not need to be vigorous.

Muscle Strength

Without strength training, you will lose muscle mass and strength: The average American loses 10 to 20 percent of muscle strength between the ages of twenty and fifty, and another 25 to 30 percent between fifty and seventy.

Strength training helps stave off changes in body composition by raising the basal metabolic rate, or the number of calories the body burns at rest. The more muscle you have, the higher your metabolic rate, the more calories you burn, and the easier it is to fight flab.

To avoid the loss of muscle, you must do strength-building exercises as well as aerobic exercise. Studies have shown that people who maintain their aerobic fitness still lose muscle mass—about one pound of muscle every two years after age twenty—if they don't diversify their workouts to include strength training.

Training Tips

- Your training weight should be 70 to 80 percent of the maximum weight you can lift while still correctly performing an exercise maneuver for a single repetition. So if the heaviest weight you can lift in a certain maneuver is fifty pounds, your training weight for that exercise would be thirty-five to forty pounds. You should be able to lift this weight eight to twelve times. Once you can lift a weight twenty times, it's time to move up to a heavier weight.
- One set of each exercise is almost as effective as multiple sets in building muscles and boosting metabolism.
- Three workouts per week is the basic recommendation for building muscle. You should, however, be able to maintain your current level of strength with two strength-training sessions a week.
- Take it slow and easy. Each repetition of an exercise should take about six seconds—two seconds for the first half of the maneuver and four for the return to the original position.
- Use good form. Doing an exercise incorrectly can cause muscle damage and injury.
- Don't hold your breath. Holding your breath can cause a dangerous rise in blood pressure, then a sudden drop when you release your breath, possibly causing light-headedness or fainting. Inhale, then exhale during the exertion phase of the movement, and inhale during the release.

Stoke Your Furnace

Your basal metabolic rate is the number of calories your body uses when it is at rest. Unless you run a marathon or exercise for a prolonged period, the basal metabolic rate accounts for most of the calories your body burns.

Your metabolic rate is influenced by your age (the older you are, the fewer calories you burn), your physical activity level (the more you exercise, the more calories you burn), and the amount of muscle you have (a pound of muscle burns more than twice as many calories as a pound of fat).

When you exercise for as little as thirty minutes, your basal metabolic rate rises by as much as 10 percent, and it can remain elevated for approximately forty-eight hours after the activity. This means that after you finish your workout, your body is burning more calories, even if you are sitting on the couch watching television.

Flexibility

Flexibility is a critical part of fitness—but one that is often overlooked. Flexibility is more than touching your toes; it involves maintaining the range of motion in your joints, which can allow you to perform your everyday activities without discomfort. It also makes you less prone to muscle strains, sprains, and tears. The only way to preserve your flexibility is to perform stretching exercises regularly. This stretching will not directly improve your IBS symptoms, but it will contribute to your overall health.

As little as ten minutes of stretching every other day can help prevent stiffness and loss of flexibility. Don't stretch "cold" muscles. Instead, stretch two or three minutes into your warm-up, just after you have broken a sweat. Stretch for two minutes before aerobic activities and ten minutes before abrupt stop-and-go activities, such as tennis or basketball. You don't need to stretch before strength training, but you should afterward. Regardless of the type of exercise you perform, after your workout stretch two minutes for every ten minutes of your workout time.

To build flexibility, bend or flex until you feel tension or slight discomfort—but not pain—and hold each stretch for twenty to sixty seconds. Do not hold your breath, and do not bounce or pulse, which can tear the connective tissue in the joints.

GETTING STARTED

No matter what your age, it's never too late to start exercising, but don't expect to overcome decades of inactivity in a couple of weeks. It took a long time to get out of shape, and it will take some time to get back in shape, so be patient with yourself. You'll start to feel the physical and emotional benefits of exercise in a few weeks, and your fitness level will continue to improve over the next few months. Studies have shown that a year of regular exercise can return the body to a fitness level of ten years earlier.

To get in shape, you will have to make a commitment to exercise regularly; sporadic exercise won't bring the rewards of fitness. Your body will adapt to the physical demands you place on it, and it will do so without injury or discomfort, if you exercise sensibly.

You can push yourself and overload your muscles in one of

three ways: by increasing the intensity of exercise (the amount of weight you lift or the speed you run), the duration of exercise (the length of time you work out), or the frequency of exercise (the number of workouts per week). As a rule of thumb, limit your overload to no more than a 10 percent increase in intensity, duration, or frequency per week to allow your body to adjust to your fitness program gradually.

Once you start exercising, keep at it. Consistency counts. If you miss a few days of exercise, don't feel guilty and throw in the towel (literally). Instead, just get back to it, but don't try to make up for lost time by increasing the intensity of your workout. In fact, if you skip exercise for one week, cut back on the intensity of your workout and gradually build up again. You start to lose aerobic conditioning and strength if you sit it out for as little as one week.

Make an appointment to exercise. Put it on your schedule and honor it as you would any other important appointment.

WARNING: *If you have coronary disease or take medications regularly, consult your doctor before starting an exercise program. Also talk to your doctor if you're a smoker, if you haven't had a checkup in more than two years, if you're more than twenty pounds overweight, or if you have a risk factor for coronary disease, such as diabetes, lung disease, hypertension, high levels of LDL cholesterol or low levels of HDL cholesterol, or a family history of early heart attack.*

EVERY LITTLE BIT HELPS

There are any number of ways to make exercise part of your daily routine.

- Park at the far end of the parking lot, rather than in the closest space.
- Take the stairs, rather than the elevator or escalator.
- Walk your child to school.
- Mow the lawn with a manual mower.
- Knead bread.
- Mop the floors.
- Rake the leaves.
- Pick up trash.
- Walk or bike to the market.
- Do housework instead of hiring help.
- Wash your car instead of using a drive-through wash.
- Put away the remote control.
- Get off the bus or subway one or two stops early and walk to your final destination.
- Stand up when you're on the phone.
- Walk around the block for a break during the workday.
- Join the company sports team; or start a team if there isn't one in your community.
- Play with your kids (or the neighbor's kids).
- Plan vacations that include exercise or activity.
- Walk on the beach.
- Dance.

After Your Workout

A sauna can be a relaxing—and beneficial—conclusion to a workout. The intense heat helps the body release toxins from the fat storage sites, cleansing the body and in turn improving IBS symptoms.

I recommend the use of low-temperature saunas because they encourage the release of oily sweat rather than watery sweat associated with high-temperature saunas. In my experience, low-temperature saunas have much more therapeutic value than the high-temperature kind.

How do low- and high-temperature saunas differ?

- Low-temperature saunas involve the use of lower temperatures: 110 to 120 degrees Fahrenheit, rather than 120 degrees and higher, as is common with high-temperature saunas.
- Sessions in a low-temperature sauna last thirty to sixty minutes, compared to ten to fifteen minutes for high-temperature saunas.

After the sauna, immediately shower with a glycerin soap such as Neutrogena, black soap, or a similar superfatted soap. This is quite important to prevent the secreted oils from being reabsorbed. A loofah or similar gentle scrub brush is recommended. In addition, a cool shower is invigorating and refreshing.

It is safe to begin your exercise program at the same time you change your diet and begin taking nutritional supplements. (Nutritional supplements are discussed in the next chapter.) Your IBS symptoms will begin to subside almost immediately after exercise, and regular workouts will help restore normal intestinal function. You will be surprised at how quickly you will experience relief from IBS—as well as the many other benefits of regular exercise.

Chapter 11

Nutritional Supplements

Imagine that you're doing everything right regarding your diet: You eat a balanced diet, filled with nutrient-rich vegetables, fruits, and whole foods. You never overeat, skip meals, or succumb to the lure of fast-food advertising. You have identified the foods that trigger your IBS and take steps to avoid them. Most importantly, you feel better than you have in years and your IBS symptoms have all but disappeared.

If you came to me as a patient, I would applaud your efforts, then recommend that you take several nutritional supplements. You cannot get all the nutrients you need from the foods you eat. For one thing, few of us actually adhere to an ideal diet all the time. Also, the body isn't always as efficient as it should be at extracting nutrients from food. (The ability to extract nutrients from foods diminishes with age.) In addition, modern-day intensive farming methods and depleted soils have reduced the nutrient content of food.

If you have IBS, you need intensive doses of several nutrients. The chronic diarrhea and constipation that plague IBS sufferers disrupt the body's ability to absorb nutrients from foods, leaving them deficient in many key nutrients. This diminished nutrition triggers a further cascade of symptoms, because the body does not have the nutrients it needs to function properly.

A chronic lack of vitamins and minerals sets the stage for disease. Nutritional deficiencies increase the toxicity of harmful bacteria because the body lacks the nutritional support to keep the bacteria in check. In addition, the detoxification process itself relies on minerals to perform the necessary metabolic functions. This lack of nutrients no doubt contributes to the fact that two out of three Americans suffers from a chronic medical problem, such as IBS.

I recommend that my patients take nutritional supplements that will help to repair the digestive system for several weeks before adding other nutrients. Until the digestive system has healed from the damage caused by IBS, the nutrients cannot be absorbed and used by the body. In addition, the nutrients can create a detoxification effect, so you should make these changes gradually. Taking too much too soon wastes money and offers no nutritional benefit. For this reason, I have divided the IBS Supplement Plan into two phases: Phase 1 for Rebuilding and Repair and Phase 2 for Building Nutrient Reserves.

PHASE 1: REBUILDING AND REPAIR (1 TO 2 WEEKS)

During the first phase of the IBS program, the goal is to strengthen the digestive system by reducing inflammation, restoring normal flora, and normalizing bowel transit time. Taking too many supplements too quickly can have undesirable side effects caused by a rapid die-off of candida or bacteria or toxic exposure caused by rapid detoxification. The following supplements help heal the digestive system, especially when used in combination with dietary changes described in chapter 7.

Vitamin C

Take 1,500 milligrams of a pure, pharmaceutical-grade nonoxidizable fully reduced and powdered vitamin C four times a day.

Vitamin C reduces inflammation, stimulates the immune system, and restores the mucous lining of the gastrointestinal tract. In addition, vitamin C creates an environment in the digestive tract that helps control the overgrowth of yeast, bacteria, and parasites.

Because the body cannot manufacture vitamin C, it must be obtained through the diet or in the form of supplements. Vitamin C deficiency can contribute to digestive problems, as well as bleeding gums, increased susceptibility to infection, joint pain, bruising, and lack of energy.

Vitamin C can be taken as buffered tablets or powders, which can be mixed with water or sparkling mineral water to make a flavored drink. I recommend the powdered version, which can be immediately absorbed and creates a stronger alkaline response in the body. (Chewable vitamin C supplements damage tooth enamel and are not the recommended form or quality.) Choose a form of vitamin C that uses buffered mineral ascorbate, such as that made by Pure Essentials® (see appendix).

While the recommended dose (1,500 milligrams four

times a day) is a good starting point for most of my patients, some people may need to adjust their dosage to maximize or minimize the effect. To find out the ideal dosage for you, see "Customizing Your Dosage of Vitamin C" on page 163.

Quercetin

Take 1,000 milligrams of quercetin and OPC four times a day, once in the morning and again at night (with the vitamin C).

The bioflavonoid quercetin helps the body utilize vitamin C. It also helps alter the digestive environment, making it hostile to yeast, bacteria, and parasites. In addition, quercetin promotes circulation, stimulates bile production, lowers cholesterol levels, and helps prevent cataracts.

The body cannot produce quercetin, so it must be supplied by the diet or supplements. Bioflavonoids (also known as flavonoids) are pigments that protect plants from free-radical damage; quercetin is a yellow-green bioflavonoid.

Look for a product containing quercetin dehydrate, which is the most bioavailable form. Other forms of quercetin are poorly assimilated by the body.

Glutamine

Take 2 grams of glutamine daily, 1 gram on an empty stomach in the morning and a second 1-gram dose on an empty stomach in the evening.

The amino acid glutamine is an essential nutrient for the treatment of IBS because it helps speed repair of the gastrointestinal lining, and it assists in the maintenance of the proper acid–alkaline balance in the body. When glutamine reserves dip too low, the body excretes excessive amounts of calcium, magnesium, potassium, and phosphorus, which push the body toward a more acidic state. In addition, the brain relies on glutamine for cerebral function and the production of neurotransmitters.

Supplemental L-glutamine can be helpful in the treatment of IBS, as well as arthritis, autoimmune diseases, connective tissue diseases, and tissue damage due to radiation treatment for cancer. It can enhance mental functioning and has been used to treat a range of problems including senility, epilepsy, depression, and schizophrenia. L-glutamine decreases sugar cravings and the desire for alcohol, and is useful for recovering alcoholics.

L-glutamine, like other amino acids, is available in multivitamin formulas, food supplements, protein mixtures, and amino acid formulas, but I recommend that it be taken in capsule form and taken separately from other supplements, foods, or protein mixtures.

Supplemental glutamine must be kept absolutely dry or it will degrade into ammonia and glutamic acid. Be aware that although the names sound similar, glutamine, glutamic acid (also sometimes called glutamate), glutathione, gluten, and monosodium glutamate are all different substances.

Acidophilus

Take two doses of freeze-dried *Lactobacillus acidophilus* three times a day with food.

The probiotic or helpful bacterium known as *L. acidophilus* produces the enzyme lactase, which helps digest lactose, a milk sugar. It also performs a number of essential functions in the body:

- It encourages the growth of beneficial bacteria in the digestive and urinary tracts; the reestablishment of microbial balance is crucial in the treatment of IBS.
- It discourages the growth of yeast and harmful bacteria, including salmonella, streptococci, *E. coli,* and staphylococci; it also has antiviral and antifungal effects.
- It helps maintain optimal intestinal pH, which, in turn, helps with complete digestion.
- It assists with digestion by producing certain digestive enzymes.
- It increases the absorption of minerals, such as calcium, magnesium, and sometimes iron.
- It produces some of the B vitamins, including biotin, niacin, folic acid, pantothenic acid, vitamin B_{12}, and vitamin B_6.
- It protects against food allergies by maintaining an optimal intestinal lining, which protects against leaky gut syndrome and development of food allergies.
- It protects against parasites, and prevents some parasites from transforming into more aggressive, disease-causing strains.

I recommend the use of *L. acidophilus* both during the repair phase and on a continuing basis. In addition to the *L. acidophilus,* the supplement should contain *bifido breve, bifido longum, L. plantarum,* and *L. rhamnosus.* (Check the bottle for the correct strains of bacteria.) The freeze-dried form is most stable and easily used by the body.

Supplement Troubleshooting

If, after one to two weeks, you still have constipation or diarrhea, make the following changes to the supplement plan:

- **Still constipated:** Double the dose of vitamin C and quercetin. Leave the glutamine and acidophilus levels the same.
- **Still have diarrhea:** Halve the dose of vitamin C and quercetin. Leave the glutamine and acidophilus levels the same.

PHASE 2: BUILDING NUTRIENT RESERVES (LIFETIME)

The second phase of the supplement program may be started when both constipation and diarrhea have been resolved. You should have daily bowel movements with an average transit time of twelve to eighteen hours; one to three bowel movements a day is normal, provided there is no diarrhea.

Amino Acid Complex

Take one dose of an amino acid complex for liver detoxification twice a day.

Follow the dosage information listed on the product you choose. The liver is the toxic filter for the entire body; it must have a chance to release these toxins and to repair itself in order to work efficiently. A comprehensive amino acid complex designed for liver detoxification will help with systemic detoxification; it also helps normalize bile and digestive functions, assists with protein synthesis, and allows the body to maintain a more alkaline level.

A good product contains the following amino acids:

- Glycine
- L-phenylalanine
- L-methionine
- L-cysteine
- L-cysteine HCI
- L-glutathione
- L-aspartate
- Choline
- Inositol
- Ascorbyl palmitate
- Calcium and magnesium co-factors

Multivitamin

Take two high-quality multivitamins twice a day.

If you have IBS, you are almost certainly deficient in a number of key nutrients. By taking a good multivitamin, you can restore your nutrient reserves, which are essential for good health.

Not all multivitamins are the same. A good multivitamin contains the following ingredients:

Optimal Multivitamin Ingredients

Nutrient	Recommended Dosage	% of RDA
Vitamin A (beta-carotene)	5,000 IU	100%
Vitamin B_1	100 mg	6,666%
Vitamin B_2	50 mg	2,941%
Vitamin B_3 (niacin)	25 mg	125%
Vitamin B_3 (niacinamide)	75 mg	375%
Vitamin B_5	100 mg	1,000%
Vitamin B_6	200 mg	10,000%
Vitamin B_{12}	200 mcg	3,333%
Folate	400 mcg	100%
Biotin	500 mcg	166%
Vitamin C	150 mg	250%
Vitamin D	400 IU	100%
Vitamin E	200 IU	667%
Vitamin K	500 mcg	625%
Potassium	99 mg	3%
Calcium	1,000 mg	100%
Magnesium	100 mg	25%
Zinc	25 mg	167%
Chromium	200 mcg	167%
Manganese	15 mg	750%
Molybdenum	100 mcg	133%
Selenium	50 mcg	71%

Other recommended, but not essential ingredients:

PABA	30 mcg	*
Octacosanol	500 mcg	*
Boron	2 mg	*
Quercetin	100 mg	*
Vanadium	100 mcg	*
L-aspartic acid	50 mg	*
Trimethylglycine	50 mg	*
Triacontanol	744 mcg	*
Hexacosanol	33 mcg	*
Tetracosanol	193 mcg	*
Citrate	59 mg	*
Fumarate	59 mg	*
Malate	59 mg	*
Succinate	59 mg	*
Vegetable fiber	170 mg	*

*No RDA available.

Ginger Tea

Drink up to four or five cups of ginger tea daily.

Common ginger has a very long history of use as a digestive stimulant in the treatment of IBS and other gastrointestinal problems. The volatile oils in dried rhizome of ginger, including gingerols, shogaols, and bisabolene, contribute to the herb's healing power. It also makes the body more alkaline and combats yeast overgrowth. Ginger is available as a fresh root (the preferred form), dried root powder, and as tablets, capsules, and prepared tea bags. If you use a commercial preparation, follow package directions.

To make a decoction, simmer one to two teaspoons of dried root powder in one cup of water for five to ten minutes. If you prefer to use fresh ginger, simmer one teaspoon of grated fresh gingerroot in one cup of water for fifteen minutes; strain before drinking.

CAUTION: *Ginger can be useful for the treatment of morning sickness, but the long-term use of ginger during pregnancy is not recommended. If you have a history of gallstones, consult your physician before taking ginger.*

The A, B, Cs of Vitamins and Minerals

Scientists have identified more than fifty different nutrients—including vitamins, essential minerals (needed in relatively large amounts), trace minerals (needed in relatively small amounts), and electrolytes. They are all necessary for human health. Vitamins and minerals function together to initiate and promote virtually every chemical and molecular reaction in the body.

- **Vitamins** are organic substances that the body needs to regulate metabolism, assist in biochemical processes, and prevent disease. Vitamins are either fat soluble or water soluble. As the name implies, fat-soluble vitamins dissolve in fat; they can be stored by the body for long periods of time and build up to toxic levels if taken in excess. Water-soluble vitamins cannot be stored and must be consumed every day or two; excess levels are eliminated in the urine.

- **Minerals** are basic elements; they cannot be manufactured or broken down by living systems. Minerals do, however, combine with vitamins, enzymes, and other substances as part of essential metabolic processes in the body.

CUSTOMIZING YOUR DOSAGE OF VITAMIN C

During Phase 1 of the program, you will be taking nutrients at a level high enough to allow the body to repair itself. Ideally, the body reaches a saturation point, after which you can shift to a lower maintenance dose. This change in dosing is particularly important for vitamin C.

While most people will respond to the recommended Phase 1 dose of vitamin C (1,500 milligrams four times a day), there are great variations among individuals' needs for vitamin C. To determine the optimal level of vitamin C for your body, you may want to perform a vitamin C flush. I recommend that you begin Phase 1 with the recommended dosages and do the flush if constipation has not resolved within two weeks.

- Dissolve ½ teaspoon (2 grams) of buffered ascorbate (a potassium, calcium, magnesium, zinc combination of vitamin C) in ½ ounce of water or juice, then drink. (You can find buffered ascorbate at a pharmacy or health food store.)
- Repeat every fifteen minutes until a watery diarrhea without stool occurs (as if you are taking an enema). If you do not flush after three hours, increase to 1 teaspoon every fifteen minutes.
- After the watery diarrhea occurs, stop consuming the ascorbate. The diarrhea is not a side effect; it means the

body has reached the point at which it cannot absorb any more ascorbate. The diarrhea has a cleansing effect on the body.

- To determine your ideal daily ascorbate requirement, figure out the total amount of ascorbate that you consumed during the flush up to the point the watery diarrhea first occurred. For example, if you consumed 8 doses of ½ teaspoon each, you would have consumed a total of 4 teaspoons (8 x ½ = 4). Your daily ascorbate requirement would be 75 percent of that total: in this case, 3 teaspoons (4 x 0.75 = 3).
- As you become healthier, your body will need less ascorbate to achieve the same saturation point. As your need for ascorbate decreases, you will notice a loosening of stool (not diarrhea). At this point, you can decrease your daily dose accordingly.

Many of my patients report a feeling of well-being after a vitamin C flush. You may repeat the procedure as often as once a week; when you know your basic flush dosage, you can complete the process at the end of the day in about one hour.

CHOOSING THE RIGHT BRAND OF SUPPLEMENTS

In order for a nutritional supplement to be effective, it must be formulated in such a way that the nutrients will be available to the body, and it should not contain any fillers or impurities. Exposés on vitamins have found that more than one out of every three brands did not dissolve in time to be of use to the body, making their bioavailability zero. In response, in 2003 the Food and Drug Administration proposed manufacturing standards for the $19 billion nutritional supplement industry to ensure ingredient and dosage accuracy and to outlaw products with dangerous contaminants. The regulations will be adopted in 2004 and phased in after that time.

It can be very difficult to choose among the twenty-four hundred vitamin brands available in the United States. Many manufacturers buy the chemicals they use in their vitamins from the same sources, but mix them with different fillers. Some manufacturers actually use ingredients that react with each other, which radically reduces their usefulness. In fact, even among the most reputable brands, only 30 to 70 percent of the nutrients are biochemically available.

Ideally, supplements should be balanced so that the body will have all the nutrients it needs to complete a metabolic function. Supplements should include the nutrients and the co-factors, which are secondary nutrients necessary for the body to use the nutrients. For example, a good amino acid formula should include calcium and magnesium as co-factors.

Purity is another problem, whether a vitamin is labeled "natural" or not. Look for pharmaceutical-quality supplements packaged with appropriate co-factors; I recommend Pure Essentials, Allergy Research, and Tyson as reliable, widely available brands. Also look for supplements that adhere to the USP (United States Pharmacopoeia) standard, which guarantees dissolvability.

Chapter 12

Putting It All Together: Thirty Days to a Healthier Digestive System

What did you have for dinner last night? How about last Thursday night? Did you remember to take your morning multivitamin? It can be difficult to keep track of the foods you eat and how you felt after eating them unless you keep a detailed food diary. In addition, it can be difficult to remember all of the items on your IBS Plan to-do list unless you outline a written plan.

This chapter will help you utilize all the information discussed in this book, and it will give you a convenient place to jot notes about your food reactions. When making notes about possible food sensitivities, refer to the list of symptoms found on page 16 for guidance.

NOTE: *Before implementing the suggestions in this book, you should have your condition assessed by a doctor to rule out the possibility that your IBS symptoms are part of a more serious illness. Chapter 3 can help you understand various diagnostic tests.*

Day 1

Diet

- Follow the Phase 1 diet (on page 78), following the basic guidelines of an 80–20 alkaline–acid balance, low-carbohydrate, no-yeast, no-dairy diet plan. Eat only those foods marked as part of the Core Diet, as described beginning on page 81.

Supplements

- Take 1,500 milligrams of powdered vitamin C four times a day.
- Take 1,000 milligrams of quercetin four times a day with the morning and evening doses of vitamin C.
- Take 2 grams of glutamine daily, 1 gram in the morning before eating and the second late in the evening before sleep.
- Take one dose of freeze-dried acidophilus three times a day with meals.

Exercise

- Practice the Intestinal Exercises found on page 138, as needed.
- Twenty to thirty minutes of aerobic exercise, with stretching.

Relaxation

- Practice ten minutes of progressive relaxation and deep breathing after meals or as needed.

Food Diary

Food Eaten	*When*	*How Much*	*How I Felt*

Day 2

Diet

- Phase 1, same as on Day 1.

Supplements

- Same as on Day 1.

Relaxation

- Same as on Day 1.

Exercise

- Practice the Intestinal Exercises found on page 138, as needed.
- Twenty to thirty minutes of weight training, with stretching.

Food Diary

Food Eaten	*When*	*How Much*	*How I Felt*

Day 3

Diet

- Phase 1, same as on Day 1.

Supplements

- Same as on Day 1.

Relaxation

- Same as on Day 1.

Exercise

- Practice the Intestinal Exercises found on page 138, as needed.
- Twenty to thirty minutes of aerobic exercise, with stretching.

Food Diary

Food Eaten	*When*	*How Much*	*How I Felt*

Day 4

Diet

- Phase 1, same as on Day 1.

Supplements

- Same as on Day 1.

Relaxation

- Practice ten minutes of progressive relaxation and deep breathing after meals or as needed.
- Consider adding meditation to your daily relaxation routine.

Exercise

- Practice the Intestinal Exercises found on page 138, as needed.
- Twenty to thirty minutes of weight training, with stretching.

Food Diary

Food Eaten	*When*	*How Much*	*How I Felt*

Day 5

Diet

- Phase 1, same as on Day 1.

Supplements

- Same as on Day 1.

Relaxation

- Same as on Day 4.

Exercise

- Practice the Intestinal Exercises found on page 138, as needed.
- Twenty to thirty minutes of aerobic exercise, with stretching.

Food Diary

Food Eaten	*When*	*How Much*	*How I Felt*

Day 6

Diet

- Phase 1, same as on Day 1.

Supplements

- Same as on Day 1.

Relaxation

- Same as on Day 4.

Exercise

- Practice the Intestinal Exercises found on page 138, as needed.
- Twenty to thirty minutes of weight training, with stretching.

Food Diary

Food Eaten	*When*	*How Much*	*How I Felt*

Day 7

Diet

- Phase 1, same as on Day 1.

Supplements

- Same as on Day 1.

Relaxation

- Same as on Day 4.

Exercise

- Rest.

Food Diary

Food Eaten	*When*	*How Much*	*How I Felt*

Day 8

Diet

- Phase 1, same as on Day 1.

Supplements

- Same as on Day 1.

Relaxation

- Same as on Day 4.

Exercise

- Practice the Intestinal Exercises found on page 138, as needed.
- Twenty to thirty minutes of aerobic exercise, with stretching.

Food Diary

Food Eaten	*When*	*How Much*	*How I Felt*

DAY 9

Diet

- Phase 1, same as on Day 1.

Supplements

- Same as on Day 1.

Relaxation

- Practice ten minutes of progressive relaxation and deep breathing after meals or as needed.
- Consider adding meditation to your daily relaxation routine.
- If you continue to have IBS symptoms, consider setting up an appointment with a hypnotist or biofeedback expert to learn how to use your mind to change your body's physiological response.

Exercise

- Practice the Intestinal Exercises found on page 138, as needed.
- Twenty to thirty minutes of weight training, with stretching.

Food Diary

Food Eaten	*When*	*How Much*	*How I Felt*

Day 10

Diet

- Phase 1, same as on Day 1.

Supplements

- Same as on Day 1.

Relaxation

- Same as on Day 9.

Exercise

- Practice the Intestinal Exercises found on page 138, as needed.
- Twenty to thirty minutes of aerobic exercise, with stretching.

Food Diary

Food Eaten	*When*	*How Much*	*How I Felt*

DAY 11

Diet
- Phase 1, same as on Day 1.

Supplements
- Same as on Day 1.

Relaxation
- Same as on Day 9.

Exercise
- Practice the Intestinal Exercises found on page 138, as needed.
- Twenty to thirty minutes of weight training, with stretching.

Food Diary

Food Eaten	*When*	*How Much*	*How I Felt*

DAY 12

Diet
- Phase 1, same as on Day 1.

Supplements
- Same as on Day 1.

Relaxation

- Same as on Day 9.

Exercise

- Practice the Intestinal Exercises found on page 138, as needed.
- Twenty to thirty minutes of aerobic exercise, with stretching.

Food Diary

Food Eaten	*When*	*How Much*	*How I Felt*

DAY 13

Diet

- Phase 1, same as on Day 1.

Supplements

- Same as on Day 1.

Relaxation

- Same as on Day 9.

Exercise

- Practice the Intestinal Exercises found on page 138, as needed.

- Twenty to thirty minutes of weight training, with stretching.

Food Diary

Food Eaten	*When*	*How Much*	*How I Felt*

Day 14

Diet

- Phase 1, same as on Day 1.

Supplements

- If the bowels have normalized (no diarrhea, no constipation, and a transit time of twelve to eighteen hours), continue taking the other supplements (as outlined for Day 1) and add:
  - Two doses of amino acid complex for liver detoxification twice a day
  - One multivitamin complex in the morning and one in the evening
  - Up to four or five cups of ginger tea, as desired
- If you still have constipation, double the dose of quercetin and vitamin C until your bowels normalize.
- If you still have diarrhea, cut the dose of vitamin C in half.

Relaxation

- Same as on Day 9.

Exercise

- Practice the Intestinal Exercises found on page 138, as needed.
- Rest.

Food Diary

Food Eaten	*When*	*How Much*	*How I Felt*

DAY 15

Diet

- Begin Phase 2 of the IBS diet (on page 80), while continuing to follow the Core Diet. Add one food not listed on the Core Diet and watch for food reactions.

Supplements

- Same as on Day 14.

Relaxation

- Practice ten minutes of progressive relaxation and deep breathing after meals or as needed.
- Consider adding meditation to your daily relaxation routine.

- If you continue to have IBS symptoms, consider setting up an appointment with a hypnotist or biofeedback expert to learn how to use your mind to change your body's physiological response.
- Consider adding visualization to your relaxation program for variety.

Exercise

- Practice the Intestinal Exercises found on page 138, as needed.
- Twenty to thirty minutes of aerobic exercise, with stretching.

Food Diary

Food Eaten	*When*	*How Much*	*How I Felt*

Day 16

Diet

- Phase 2, same as on Day 15.
- Watch for food reactions.

Supplements

- Same as on Day 14.

Relaxation

- Same as on Day 15.

Exercise

- Practice the Intestinal Exercises found on page 138, as needed.
- Twenty to thirty minutes of weight training, with stretching.

Food Diary

Food Eaten	*When*	*How Much*	*How I Felt*

Day 17

Diet

- Phase 2, same as on Day 15.
- Add a food not permitted on the Core Diet.

Supplements

- Same as on Day 14.

Relaxation

- Same as on Day 15.

Exercise

- Practice the Intestinal Exercises found on page 138, as needed.
- Twenty to thirty minutes of aerobic exercise, with stretching.

Food Diary

Food Eaten	*When*	*How Much*	*How I Felt*

DAY 18

Diet

- Phase 2, same as on Day 15.
- Watch for food reactions.

Supplements

- Same as on Day 14.

Relaxation

- Same as on Day 15.

Exercise

- Practice the Intestinal Exercises found on page 138, as needed.
- Twenty to thirty minutes of weight training, with stretching.

Food Diary

Food Eaten	*When*	*How Much*	*How I Felt*

Day 19

Diet

- Phase 2, same as on Day 15.
- Add another food not permitted on the Core Diet.

Supplements

- Same as on Day 14.

Relaxation

- Same as on Day 15.

Exercise

- Practice the Intestinal Exercises found on page 138, as needed.
- Twenty to thirty minutes of aerobic exercise, with stretching.

Food Diary

Food Eaten	*When*	*How Much*	*How I Felt*

Day 20

Diet

- Phase 2, same as on Day 15.
- Watch for food reactions.

Supplements

- Same as on Day 14.

Relaxation

- Same as on Day 15.

Exercise

- Practice the Intestinal Exercises found on page 138, as needed.
- Twenty to thirty minutes of weight training, with stretching.

Food Diary

Food Eaten	*When*	*How Much*	*How I Felt*

Day 21

Diet

- Phase 2, same as on Day 15.
- Add another food not permitted on the Core Diet.
- If you remain in Phase 1 because your IBS symptoms have persisted, try a liquid-only cleansing diet for two or three days, as described on page 92.

Supplements

- If bowels have normalized, continue taking the same supplements (see Day 14).
- If you still have constipation, try a vitamin C flush, then base your dosage of vitamin C on the results of the flush (described on page 163).

Relaxation

- Same as on Day 15.

Exercise

- Practice the Intestinal Exercises found on page 138, as needed.
- Rest.

Food Diary

Food Eaten	*When*	*How Much*	*How I Felt*

Day 22

Diet

- Phase 2, same as on Day 15.
- Watch for food reactions.

Supplements

- Same as on Day 14.

Relaxation

- Same as on Day 15.

Exercise

- Practice the Intestinal Exercises found on page 138, as needed.
- Twenty to thirty minutes of aerobic exercise, with stretching.

Food Diary

Food Eaten	*When*	*How Much*	*How I Felt*

Day 23

Diet

- Phase 2, same as on Day 15.
- Add another food not permitted on the Core Diet and watch for food reactions.

Supplements

- Same as on Day 14.

Relaxation

- Same as on Day 15.

Exercise

- Practice the Intestinal Exercises found on page 138, as needed.
- Twenty to thirty minutes of weight training, with stretching.

Food Diary

Food Eaten	*When*	*How Much*	*How I Felt*

Day 24

Diet

- Phase 2, same as on Day 15.
- Watch for food reactions.

Supplements

- Same as on Day 14.

Relaxation

- Same as on Day 15.

Exercise

- Practice the Intestinal Exercises found on page 138, as needed.
- Twenty to thirty minutes of aerobic exercise, with stretching.

Food Diary

Food Eaten	*When*	*How Much*	*How I Felt*

Day 25

Diet

- Phase 2, same as on Day 15.
- Add another food not permitted on the Core Diet and watch for food reactions.

Supplements

- Same as on Day 14.

Relaxation

- Same as on Day 15.

Exercise

- Practice the Intestinal Exercises found on page 138, as needed.

- Twenty to thirty minutes of weight training, with stretching.

Food Diary

Food Eaten	*When*	*How Much*	*How I Felt*

DAY 26

Diet
- Phase 2, same as on Day 15.
- Watch for food reactions.

Supplements
- Same as on Day 14.

Relaxation
- Same as on Day 15.

Exercise
- Practice the Intestinal Exercises found on page 138, as needed.
- Twenty to thirty minutes of aerobic exercise, with stretching.

Food Diary

Food Eaten	*When*	*How Much*	*How I Felt*

Day 27

Diet

- Phase 2, same as on Day 15.
- Add another food not permitted in the Core Diet and watch for food reactions.

Supplements

- Same as on Day 14.

Relaxation

- Same as on Day 15.

Exercise

- Practice the Intestinal Exercises found on page 138, as needed.
- Twenty to thirty minutes of weight training, with stretching.

Food Diary

Food Eaten	*When*	*How Much*	*How I Felt*

Day 28

Diet

- Phase 2, same as on Day 15.
- Watch for food reactions.

Supplements

- Same as on Day 14.

Relaxation

- Same as on Day 15.

Exercise

- Practice the Intestinal Exercises found on page 138, as needed.
- Rest.

Food Diary

Food Eaten	*When*	*How Much*	*How I Felt*

Day 29

Diet

- Phase 2, same as on Day 15.
- Add another food not permitted on the Core Diet and watch for food reactions.

Supplements

- Same as on Day 14.

Relaxation

- Same as on Day 15.

Exercise

- Practice the Intestinal Exercises found on page 138, as needed.
- Twenty to thirty minutes of aerobic exercise, with stretching.

Food Diary

Food Eaten	*When*	*How Much*	*How I Felt*

Day 30

Diet

- Phase 2, same as on Day 15.
- Watch for food reactions.

Supplements

- Same as on Day 14.

Relaxation

- Same as on Day 15.

Exercise

- Practice the Intestinal Exercises found on page 138, as needed.
- Twenty to thirty minutes of aerobic exercise, with stretching.

Food Diary

Food Eaten	*When*	*How Much*	*How I Felt*

And Beyond

Diet

- Continue to add additional vegetables, grains, oils, meats, and other foods from the alkaline list. Watch for food reactions for forty-eight hours before adding a new food.
- Over time, begin adding acidic foods and testing for food reactions.
- Maintain the 80–20 alkaline–acid balance for three to

six months; shift to the 60–40 alkaline–acid balance at that point and maintain this ratio on an ongoing basis.

Supplements

- Continue taking supplements as recommended.

Relaxation

- Consider taking a yoga or massage class to learn to reach deeper states of relaxation.

Exercise

- Continue with aerobic exercise and weight training three times a week each; gradually increase the intensity of your workout to build strength and endurance.

Food Diary

- Continue to keep your food diary until you are free of IBS symptoms. If you continue to have IBS symptoms, bring your food diary with you to your next doctor's visit and discuss the issue.
- Many of my patients continue to keep food diaries on an ongoing basis because the process of writing down what they eat makes them feel more accountable for their food choices.

Chapter 13

Gluten Intolerance (Celiac Disease)

Irritable bowel syndrome is an exasperating condition, but not a medically dangerous one. On the other hand, celiac disease, a disorder in which the body cannot digest gluten, is both difficult to live with and potentially debilitating for some people. Celiac disease can cause serious damage to the small intestine, and it can interfere with the digestion of nutrients. Unfortunately, IBS and celiac disease share many of the same symptoms, causing doctors to misdiagnose the condition and dismiss it as IBS. For this reason, I recommend that anyone with IBS be tested for celiac disease using a simple saliva or blood test.

Celiac disease can appear at any time in a person's life, from infancy to old age. The condition is sometimes diagnosed in infants, toddlers, and children when they fail to grow, experience chronic vomiting, or develop a bloated abdomen. Children may also exhibit severe irritability, learning disabilities, and other behavioral problems.

Celiac disease also may present itself in less obvious ways, including behavior changes such as irritability or depression, stomach upset, joint pain, muscle cramps, skin rash, mouth sores, and tingling in your legs. The classic symptoms include:

- Abdominal cramping
- Intestinal gas
- Bloating
- Chronic diarrhea, constipation, or both
- Oily stools
- Anemia (due to nutrient deficiency)
- Weight loss with large appetite

Other, less common symptoms include:
- Dental enamel defects
- Osteoporosis
- Bone and joint pain
- Fatigue
- Depression
- Infertility
- Tingling in the legs

While you can overcome irritable bowel syndrome, you must learn how to live with celiac disease. Celiac disease—also called gluten intolerance, celiac sprue, and gluten sensitive enteropathy (GSE)—is a lifelong digestive disorder that requires medical attention.

WHO IS AT RISK?

Celiac disease only affects people who are genetically susceptible. Many people experience the symptoms of celiac disease, however, and assume they have IBS and other digestive disorders. In fact, celiac disease is considered the most underdiagnosed common disease today, affecting as many as 1 out of every 130 people in the United States. According to a February 2003 issue of the journal *Archives of Internal Medicine,* a study of more than 4,000 people with no known genetic risk factors or symptoms of celiac disease found about 1 in 133 had the disorder. Among people with a close relative (sibling, child, or parent) with celiac, 1 in 22 had the condition; among those with a second-degree relative (grandparent, aunt, uncle, or cousin) with celiac, 1 in 39 had celiac disease. More important to IBS sufferers, the study found that 1 in 56 people with classical gastrointestinal symptoms (such as those for IBS) had celiac disease. The researchers based their findings on a blood test to identify antibodies in the blood, followed by a biopsy of lesions in the small intestine.

Many people have a genetic susceptibility to celiac disease, but the disease lies dormant until a triggering event occurs, such as surgery, viral infection, severe emotional stress, pregnancy, or childbirth. For reasons that are not well understood, these physical and emotional traumas can activate celiac disease in vulnerable people.

Celiac disease occurs most often in Caucasians, especially Irish and Scandinavians. It is rare among Asians, people of Jewish heritage, and African Americans. It is frequently associated with blood group O and occasionally in type A blood.

THE GLUTEN RESPONSE

Celiac disease is triggered by certain proteins found in wheat, spelt, triticale, kamut, rye, oats, barley, teff, amaranth, and quinoa (in descending order). When a person with celiac disease consumes gluten proteins, the food stimulates an autoimmune response that inflames the intestines and weakens the villi, tiny hairlike projections found in the lining of the small intestine that produce digestive enzymes and absorb nutrients in food. Over time, the villi flatten, shrink, and disappear.

The inevitable result of damaged villi is the poor absorption of nutrients, including proteins, carbohydrates, fats, vitamins, minerals, and water. Left untreated, many people with celiac disease can develop life-threatening malnutrition and other medical problems. Long-term conditions that can result from untreated celiac disease include iron deficiency anemia, osteoporosis, vitamin K deficiency associated with risk of hemorrhaging, vitamin and mineral deficiencies caused by malabsorption, central and peripheral nervous system disorders, abnormal spinal cord development, night blindness, pancreatic insufficiency, and lactose intolerance. In rare cases, the disease can cause encephalopthy (a toxic brain condition caused by vitamin B deficiency) and cancer of the small intestine.

Fortunately, many of these complications can be reduced or avoided by adhering to a strict gluten-free diet. This does not mean simply avoiding breads, cereals, and pastas; people with celiac disease must avoid all foods that contain any traces of gluten proteins, including processed foods to which gluten has been added. I have had patients who were so sensitive to gluten that they reacted to a spoon that inadvertently had touched cereal in another family member's bowl and then been placed in the patient's mouth with traces of food on it.

The Link to Dermatitis Herpetiformis

Dermatitis herpetiformis (DH) is a skin condition associated with celiac disease. It is characterized by blistering, intensely itchy patches of skin located on pressure points, such as the elbows, knees, and buttocks; the rash typically follows a symmetrical distribution. The eruptions, which resemble the early stages of a pimple, often develop into an intensely itchy, watery blister. People with DH often suffer damage to their gastrointestinal tract similar to those with celiac disease. For relief of their symptoms, people with DH must also follow a gluten-free diet.

DIAGNOSING CELIAC DISEASE

Fortunately, diagnosing celiac disease is fairly straightforward. First, patients are screened using a saliva or blood test to look for gluten antibodies in the blood. If antibodies are present, some patients confirm the test with a biopsy of a tissue sample taken from the small intestine. The biopsy shows the malformation of the villi, as well as a reduction in several important digestive enzymes.

In addition, the diagnosis is confirmed if a patient's overall health improves and his or her gastrointestinal symptoms disappear after eliminating gluten from the diet. Some doctors recommend a second small-bowel biopsy at the three-month follow-up to check on the progress of healing; I usually recommend that my patients adhere to a strict no-gluten diet without undergoing another invasive procedure.

If you plan to undergo a diagnostic test for gluten sensitivity, do not eliminate gluten from your diet before the test. Specific antibody blood tests are used to identify celiac disease, but you must be consuming gluten for the antibodies to be present.

TREATING CELIAC DISEASE

The only treatment for celiac disease is simple, but very difficult: You must scrupulously avoid gluten for the rest of your life. When gluten is removed from the diet, the small intestine will begin to heal within the first week. Full recovery, however, may take three to six months. (In rare cases, it may take up to eighteen to twenty-four months.)

I recommend that anyone with celiac disease work with a dietician to design a diet plan. Nutritional counseling is vital, because overcoming this condition requires reading every label, even on apparently innocent products such as chewing gum, medications, and vitamins. People with celiac disease should also be monitored by a gastroenterologist or other physician familiar with the disease.

People with celiac disease cannot "cheat" on their diet without short-term consequences (diarrhea and abdominal pain) as well as dire long-term consequences (a much higher risk of osteoporosis and other bone diseases, gastrointestinal cancers, and malnutrition, to name a few). Going on and off a gluten-free diet also increases your risk of malnutrition and other complications.

LIVING WITH CELIAC DISEASE

Getting used to your new diet can be difficult and frustrating. Learning what foods you can and cannot eat may take several months, during which time you may make some mistakes. You also may crave foods that you're no longer allowed to eat. But don't give up. With time, you can learn to adjust to a gluten-free diet.

You should follow the counsel of your personal dietician, but the following can give you a general guide of which foods are allowed, and which are not.

Foods You Can Eat

- Grains: Wild rice, buckwheat, millet, sorghum.
- Gluten-free flours, such as those made from ground chestnuts and other nongrains.
- Meats (not breaded or marinated).
- Fruits (all).
- Vegetables (all).
- Any ready-made product labeled "gluten-free."

For More Information

Members of a local or national celiac disease support group also can be helpful in pointing out foods that are safe to eat. To assist you when shopping, some national support groups have published books or brochures that list manufactured and commercially produced grocery items that don't contain gluten. You can get copies of these shopping guides by contacting the Celiac Sprue Association (listed in the resources section in the back of this book).

Foods You Cannot Eat

- Grains: Wheat (wheat flour, white flour, wheat bran, wheat germ, farina, wheat starch, graham flour, semolina, durum), barley, rye, oats (oat flour, oat bran, oatmeal), amaranth, bulgur, kamut, kasha, matzo meal, quinoa, spelt, teff, triticale. (Amaranth, buckwheat, and quinoa are gluten-free as grown, but they're often combined with other grains during harvesting and processing; you're better off not eating them unless you can be sure of their source.)
- Distilled vinegars, unless identified as gluten-free.
- Many processed foods in which gluten can be found, such as cold cuts, soups, soy sauces, and many low- or nonfat products. If you have questions about the gluten content of any specific food, contact the manufacturer and ask.

CHECK FOOD LABELS

Food labels are your lifeline to better health. Always read the food label before you purchase any product. You will have to read the label each time you buy, because a manufacturer may change a product's ingredients at any time.

The following ingredients may originate from gluten-containing grains. Don't eat foods with these ingredients unless you can verify from the manufacturer that the ingredients don't contain gluten:

- Unidentified starch.
- Modified food starch.
- Hydrolyzed vegetable protein (HVP).

- Hydrolyzed plant protein (HPP).
- Texturized vegetable protein (TVP).
- Malt and other natural flavorings.
- Brown rice syrup.
- Soy sauce or soy sauce solids.
- Mono- and diglycerides (in dry products).
- Caramel flavor.
- Maltodextrin.
- Alcohol-based extracts (such as vanilla, if alcohol is made from distilled grain).
- Distilled vinegar (distilled vinegar is usually made from grain).
- Ketchup, pickles, mayonnaise, salad dressings, barbecue sauce, and other condiments, since they usually contain distilled vinegar.
- Binders in some pharmaceutical products. (Before taking any drug, request clarification of product safety from the drug manufacturer.)
- Some lipsticks contain gluten; contact the manufacturer to find out if a particular product is gluten-free.
- Postage stamp glue, which sometimes contains gluten; use self-adhesive stamps.

DO YOUR HOMEWORK BEFORE YOU DRINK

Alcohol and vinegar that are properly distilled should not contain any harmful gluten peptides (or prolamins). Research indicates that the gluten peptide is too large to carry over in the distillation process, but many manufacturers add gluten-containing preservatives after the distillation process. Alcohols and vinegars should be carefully investigated for additives before use. Malt vinegars are not distilled and therefore not gluten-free.

You must also be aware of the risk of cross contamination when gluten-free foods come into contact with foods containing gluten. This may happen if you share a knife for spreading butter that has bread crumbs on it, use the same toaster as others, or eat deep-fried foods that are cooked in the same oil used for breaded foods.

Overlooked Foods That Often Contain Gluten

Broth	Flours	Roux
Breading	Sauces	Soup base
Croutons	Coating mixes	Self-basting poultry
Pasta	Marinades	Imitation seafood
Stuffing	Thickeners	Imitation bacon

EATING OUT

Preparing your own meals is the best way to ensure your diet is gluten-free. But this doesn't mean that you can't eat out on occasion. The following guidelines can help you have an enjoyable dining experience:

- Visit the same restaurants so that you can become familiar with their menus.
- Ask members of your support group for suggestions on restaurants that serve gluten-free food.

- Select simply prepared or fresh foods and avoid all breaded or batter-coated foods.
- Inspect your salad for crumbs from croutons or other bread products that have been removed.
- Bring your own salad dressing. Otherwise, use fresh lemon on your salad or vinegar made from apple cider, rice, or wine.
- Don't order soup. Most soups contain flour or a soup base that contains gluten.
- Avoid fried foods. They may be cooked in the same oil as foods containing gluten.
- Select baked or boiled potatoes. Hash brown potatoes may contain flour. French fries with coatings usually contain gluten.
- Avoid sauces or gravies. They may be thickened with flour.
- Avoid *au jus* (with sauce) foods. They may contain HVP.

GLUTEN-FREE COOKING

Giving up gluten doesn't mean that you have to give up breads, muffins, and other grain-based foods. A number of cookbooks offer gluten-free recipes so that you can safely enjoy all of your favorite foods. Several titles include:

- *Against the Grain* by Jax Peters Lowell (Henry Holt, 1996)
- *Cooking Gluten-Free!: A Food Lover's Collection of Chef and Family Recipes Without Gluten or Wheat* by Karen Robertson (Celiac Publishing, 2002)
- *The Gluten-Free Gourmet Cooks Fast and Healthy* by Bette Hagman and Joseph A. Murray (Owl Books, 2000)
- *Wheat-Free, Worry-Free: The Art of Happy, Healthy Gluten-Free Living* by Danna Korn (Hay House, 2002)

Gluten-Free Flour Substitutes

You may also be able to adapt some of your favorite recipes by making a few substitutions. For 1 tablespoon of wheat flour, substitute one of the following:

- 1½ teaspoons cornstarch
- 1½ teaspoons potato starch
- 1½ teaspoons arrowroot starch
- 1½ teaspoons rice flour
- 2 teaspoons quick-cooking tapioca

For 1 cup of wheat flour, substitute one of these:

- 1 cup corn flour
- ¾ cup plain cornmeal, coarse
- 1 cup plain cornmeal, fine
- ⅝ cup potato flour
- ¾ cup rice flour

When using substitute starches and flours, you may find that the recipe turns out best if you bake the food longer and at a lower temperature. You may need to experiment a bit to find the right length of time and temperature setting. For more satisfactory baked products, combine different substitutes. For instance, if your recipe calls for 2 cups of wheat flour, you might use ⅝ cup of potato flour and ¾ cup of rice flour.

Chapter 14

When It Isn't IBS: Understanding Other Digestive Disorders

You know there's something wrong—your chronic IBS symptoms serve as a constant reminder—but you aren't sure what's going on in your digestive system. You suffer from the classic symptoms of IBS, but could it be something else? Could you have a more serious digestive problem?

The answer, unfortunately, is yes. The vague symptoms of IBS often overlap the symptoms of other more dangerous medical problems. Without conducting diagnostic tests, even the most experienced doctors may find it difficult to differentiate between IBS and other digestive disorders, such as colitis, intestinal cancer, or chronic pancreatitis.

Of course, if you suffer from IBS, the solution is to have your condition assessed by a doctor to rule out serious illness. Diarrhea, bloating, and abdominal pain can be hallmarks of any number of conditions, and you need to be sure that you do not suffer from an illness with serious health consequences that demands medical attention.

This chapter lists several digestive problems with some

symptoms that resemble those of IBS. While many of the conditions do have symptoms that might distinguish them from IBS, there is sufficient overlap that some people might mistake one illness for another. For this reason, I encourage you to visit a doctor to rule out these conditions before following the IBS program described here.

CROHN'S DISEASE

Crohn's disease involves inflammation of any part of the gastrointestinal tract from the mouth to the anus; the most common location of the inflammation is the lower part of the small intestine (the ileum) and the large intestine (the colon).

The symptoms of Crohn's disease include:

- Chronic diarrhea
- Abdominal pain, usually on the right side (sometimes Crohn's disease is called the right-sided disease)
- Fatigue
- Fever
- Weight loss
- Rectal bleeding caused by fissures (cracks in the anal area), fistulas (abnormal openings that connect the bowel and bladder to the skin surface near the anus), and abscesses (sacs filled with pus)
- Feeling of fullness on the right side of the abdomen

While the diarrhea and abdominal pain resemble symptoms of IBS, if you experience the other symptoms, you should contact your doctor immediately. Crohn's disease can be diagnosed using colonoscopy or endoscopy, depending on the location of the inflammation.

The symptoms of Crohn's disease may subside, only to recur months or years later. In severe and lingering cases, Crohn's disease can lead to serious infections that can permanently damage the digestive system and spread to other organs.

Because Crohn's disease is similar to ulcerative colitis, the two disorders are grouped together as inflammatory bowel disease (IBD). The goal of treatment should be to eliminate the inflammatory response to permit healing of the intestinal tissue. Food allergies can exacerbate symptoms of Crohn's disease; it is important to identify and avoid allergenic foods. The IBS Program presented in this book can help stabilize the digestive system and reduce intestinal inflammation, but a patient with Crohn's disease should be under the care of a medical professional.

COLITIS

Colitis (also known as ulcerative colitis) involves inflammation of the large intestine or colon. Symptoms of colitis include:

- Diarrhea
- Abdominal cramping
- Rectal bleeding
- Blood and mucus in the stools
- Joint pain
- Skin sores or rashes

Colitis is similar to Crohn's disease; the primary differences are that Crohn's disease occurs deeper within the intestinal wall, and it can occur throughout the digestive system. While some of the symptoms overlap in colitis and IBS, bleeding is not a symptom of IBS and should be a clear sign that you need to see a doctor.

During bouts of colitis, water, minerals, and nutrients are not well absorbed by the body, leading to weight loss, dehydration, anemia, and fatigue. Although the recommendations in this book can also help relieve the symptoms of colitis, anyone who has colitis should receive care from a medical professional.

COLON CANCER

When digestive problems first occur, many people fear the worst: cancer. Although cancer isn't the cause of most gastrointestinal problems, these fears are not completely unfounded, since the symptoms of IBS overlap the symptoms of some gastrointestinal cancers, especially in the early stages. For this reason, when IBS symptoms first appear, a doctor should assess your overall health to rule out cancer, as well as other more serious health problems.

Cancer can develop anywhere in the digestive tract, but most gastrointestinal cancers occur in the colon and the rectum, where the stool moves more slowly and toxins linger. The following list includes several common types of gastrointestinal cancer and their warning signs:

- **Cancer of the esophagus:** Difficulty swallowing, blood in vomit or stool, weight loss, chest pain.

- **Cancer of the stomach:** Upper abdominal pain, nausea and vomiting, loss of appetite, feeling full after eating only a moderate amount, blood in vomit or stool.

- **Cancer of the small intestine:** Cramps, bloating, nausea and vomiting, blood in stool, weight loss.

• **Cancer of the gallbladder:** Yellowing of skin and eyes (jaundice), abdominal pain, nausea, fatigue, weight loss.

• **Cancer of the liver:** Abdominal pain, weight loss, abdominal swelling, yellowing of skin and eyes (jaundice).

• **Cancer of the pancreas:** Abdominal pain, weight loss, yellowing of skin and eyes (jaundice).

• **Cancer of the colon and rectum:** Blood in stool, change in bowel habits, abdominal pain, weight loss.

No one knows for certain how a normal cell becomes cancerous. A number of factors, including lifestyle, environment, and heredity, may be responsible. Oncologists believe that most people have dormant genes that can produce cancer cells, and that these genes do not cause problems until they're activated by an outside agent, such as an infection, tobacco, pollutants, or some sort of irritant to the body.

Colorectal cancer (cancer of the colon and rectum) is the second most common cause of cancer death in both men and women. When detected and treated early, digestive cancers are often highly curable. Unfortunately, the symptoms of gastrointestinal cancers tend to be so vague that the cancer is not diagnosed until it has reached an advanced stage. In addition, many people do not have regular screening tests, which can detect the cancer at its earliest stages.

Talk to your doctor about regular health screenings for colorectal cancer, as well as other types of cancer. I recommend colonoscopy every ten years after age fifty for people with no family history of colon cancer, with an annual fecal occult and sigmoidoscopy every five years. If a person has one immediate family member who developed colon cancer before age sixty, I recommend the first colonoscopy at age forty. If a person has two immediate family members with colon cancer before age sixty, a colonoscopy should be performed every three to five years.

DIVERTICULITIS AND DIVERTICULOSIS

At birth, the intestinal tract is a smooth, muscular tube. Over time, that smooth wall weakens and develops tiny pockets or pouches known as diverticula. (Each pouch is called a *diverticulum,* from Latin words meaning "a small diversion from the normal path"; *diverticula* refers to more than one diverticulum.)

Diverticula can form anywhere, including the throat, esophagus, stomach, and small intestine, but by far the most common site is the left-side large intestine (the descending and sigmoid colon), because this is the narrowest segment of the colon. Due to its size and position, this stretch of the colon develops the highest internal pressure, leaving it most vulnerable to diverticula. The problem can be exacerbated by a low-fiber diet high in refined sugars.

By age forty-five, about 40 percent of Americans have diverticula, and this percentage increases with age. Many people do not know they have diverticula, because they do not have any symptoms.

Diverticulitis occurs when the diverticula become infected and inflamed. The symptoms of diverticulitis include:

- Fever
- Lower abdominal pain (typically on the lower left side; the pain may be intermittent and vary in intensity)

- A lump or mass of impacted bowel (typically on the lower left side of the abdomen)
- Abdominal tenderness

Diverticulitis often starts when a small piece of food gets stuck in the pouch, giving bacteria a chance to breed. It also can occur when a small tear develops in a diverticulum, leading to infection. When infections fester, pus can collect and form an abscess. Typically, these infections resolve themselves in a few days, but in rare cases the infection spreads and bursts open the wall of the colon, causing a life-threatening infection of the abdominal cavity (peritonitis).

The diagnosis of diverticulitis can be confirmed by a CT scan or a conventional X-ray of the colon wall. In addition, the white blood count is often elevated, indicating infection. Diverticulitis is a condition that should be managed and monitored by your health care professional.

GASTROESOPHAGEAL REFLUX DISEASE (GERD)

An occasional episode of heartburn is nothing to worry about, but an estimated one out of every ten Americans suffers heartburn regularly, even daily. Frequent heartburn is the defining symptom of gastroesophageal reflux disease (GERD), a condition that deserves medical attention. While the symptoms of GERD do not directly resemble those of IBS, many people with GERD also suffer from IBS. Some people who have both conditions fail to appreciate the importance of treating GERD because they are focused on their IBS symptoms.

When you eat, food travels down your esophagus to the lower esophageal sphincter (LES), a muscular valve that separates the lower esophagus and stomach. This valve is supposed to open long enough to allow food to enter the stomach; then it is supposed to squeeze closed. When the valve doesn't close tightly, stomach acid washes back up the esophagus, a condition known as reflux. The acid can wash all the way to the upper esophagus, creating a sour, burning taste in the mouth.

Over time, the acid can damage the lining of the esophagus, causing inflammation known as esophagitis. This inflammation can narrow the esophagus, producing bleeding or difficulty swallowing.

The symptoms of GERD include:

- Frequent heartburn
- Chest pain after eating or at night
- Acid reflux
- Chronic cough
- Wheezing
- Hoarseness
- Frequent throat clearing
- Feeling a lump in the throat
- Chronic sore throat
- Difficulty swallowing
- Blood in the stool or vomit

While anyone can develop GERD, the condition does occur more frequently in people with certain risk factors. These include being overweight, having an immediate family member with the condition, smoking, consuming excessive alcohol, or being pregnant. It also occurs more often in people who have asthma, diabetes, peptic ulcer, delayed stomach emptying, connective tissue disorders, and Zollinger-Ellison syndrome (a condition in which your stomach produces extremely high amounts of acid).

Many medications can contribute to GERD by relaxing the esophageal sphincter. For example, GERD can be caused by dicyclomine (Bentyl), a medication for spastic colon; aminophylline (Theodur) for asthma; propranolol (Inderal) for hypertension and angina; diltiazem (Cardizem) for hypertension; verapamil (Calan) for hypertension; and isosorbide (Isordil) for angina.

GERD can lead to serious health problems. If you let the symptoms go, complications may arise, including:

- **Esophageal narrowing (stricture):** This narrowing of the esophagus due to a buildup of scar tissue occurs in about 10 percent of people with GERD.

- **Ulcer:** Stomach acid erodes the tissue in the esophagus, causing an open sore to form.

- **Barrett's esophagus:** The color of the tissue in the lower esophagus changes from pink to salmon. In a process called metaplasia, the cells change and begin to resemble the cells in the small intestine. This condition is associated with an increased risk of esophageal cancer. About 5 percent of people with GERD develop Barrett's esophagus; this leaves a person 30 to 125 times more likely to develop esophageal cancer than the general population.

If you experience heartburn at least twice a week for several weeks, or your symptoms seem to be getting worse, see your doctor. The IBS Program presented in this book can make a dramatic improvement in symptoms of GERD. I recommend that you follow the IBS Program in addition to consulting a physician if you have symptoms of GERD.

PANCREATITIS

Pancreatitis is an inflammation of the pancreas, the large gland that rests horizontally behind the stomach. The pancreas secretes digestive juices into the first part of the small intestine and insulin into the bloodstream. In some cases, the digestive enzymes in the pancreas leak out of their ducts and damage the pancreas, causing inflammation and bleeding in the pancreas and surrounding tissue.

Pancreatitis can occur with no apparent cause, but it usually follows a physical injury to the upper abdomen, gallbladder disease, or excessive alcohol use. Pancreatitis can be acute or chronic.

Symptoms of acute pancreatitis include:

- Nausea
- Vomiting
- High fever
- Difficulty breathing
- Abdominal bruising from internal bleeding

Chronic pancreatitis tends to be much less obvious, and it is more apt to be confused with IBS. Symptoms often go undetected for many years. Symptoms of chronic pancreatitis include:

- Periodic mild to moderate abdominal pain (though some people do not experience any pain)
- Nausea
- Vomiting
- Fever
- Bloating and gas

With chronic pancreatitis, consuming alcohol or eating large meals can make symptoms worse.

Most cases of acute pancreatitis resolve themselves without complications, but chronic pancreatitis often causes permanent damage to the pancreas, interfering with the organ's ability to produce digestive enzymes and to monitor blood sugar levels. The result can be poor absorption of nutrients (especially fats), causing weight loss and passage of loose, oily stools. Many people with chronic pancreatitis develop diabetes after their insulin-producing cells are destroyed.

Once again, pancreatitis—in both the acute and chronic forms—should be treated by a physician. With proper medical care, you should be able to avoid some of the long-term problems associated with damage to the pancreas.

PARASITES

Don't assume that parasitic infections only happen to people who travel overseas. They are far more common than most people realize, and they may cause cramping, diarrhea, and other symptoms that mimic those of IBS. As discussed throughout the book, the IBS Program presented here will help restore balanced gastrointestinal flora, which can both prevent and eradicate parasites in many cases.

A parasite lives off a host. Mild infections can create chronic symptoms that last months or years; acute infections typically create serious symptoms that demand immediate attention. Common symptoms of parasitic infection include:

- Watery diarrhea
- Intestinal cramping

- Fever
- Fatigue
- Bloating and gas
- Altered bowel habits
- Abdominal pain

Because the symptoms of parasitic infection resemble those of IBS and other digestive disorders, you should consult a physician who can do the tests necessary to accurately diagnose your condition and rule out a parasitic infection.

Left untreated, parasitic infections can cause an inflammation of the intestinal lining, leading to food allergies and problems with digestion. When the parasites embed themselves in the intestinal wall, they release toxins that can cause chronic fatigue and compromise overall health.

Conventional doctors often recommend a onetime stool sample when looking for parasites, but these tests tend to be very inaccurate. Patients with bowel problems should be tested for a wide array of parasites, including worms, bacteria, fungi, and amebae. The tests should follow an intestinal purge (such as a vitamin C flush—see page 163), so that the stool will include organisms residing high up in the intestinal lining. Research has shown that stool samples are only 30 to 40 percent accurate when done without a purge, and as much as 90 percent accurate when performed after an intestinal purge. Ask your doctor about appropriate testing.

PEPTIC ULCERS

At some point in their lives, 5 to 10 percent of Americans develop a peptic ulcer, or an open sore in the digestive tract. Ulcers located in the lining of the stomach are called gastric ulcers (gastritis); those located in the beginning of the small intestine are called duodenal ulcers (duodenitis). Ulcers in either location are called peptic, named for the digestive enzyme pepsin, which breaks down protein.

The symptoms of peptic ulcers include:

- Burning or dull, gnawing pain under the rib cage; the pain may come and go for days or weeks.
- Dissipation of pain after eating (because food helps neutralize the acid).

Left untreated, peptic ulcers can cause internal bleeding; they also can eat a hole through the wall of the stomach or small intestine, putting you at risk of serious infection. Additionally, ulcers can result in scar tissue that obstructs the passage of food through the digestive tract.

At one point, doctors believed ulcers were caused by stress and spicy foods. We now know that the bacterium *Helicobacter pylori* triggers most ulcers. This bacterium lives in the mucous layer lining the stomach and small intestine. In most people, the bacterium does not cause problems, but approximately one out of every six people infected with *H. pylori* develops an ulcer. No one knows what makes these people more susceptible to ulcers, but they may have already damaged their stomach or small intestine, creating an environment where the bacteria can more easily take over.

Infection with *H. pylori* can be diagnosed using a breath test, a blood test, or a biopsy at the time of endoscopy. The traditional treatment involves taking two antibiotics to kill the bacteria and an acid-suppressing drug for a period of two weeks. I very rarely use antibiotics in my practice to treat *H. pylori* infection; I get an excellent clinical response by following the IBS Program described in this book without the need for antibiotics. When balance is restored to the gastrointestinal tract, the underlying *H. pylori* infection has a hard time living in a normal gastrointestinal tract environment.

While *H. pylori* infection is the most common cause of peptic ulcers, other factors also play a role. These include:

- Ongoing use of nonsteroidal anti-inflammatory drugs (NSAIDs). These pain relievers can irritate or inflame the lining of your stomach and small intestine. They are available in both prescription and over-the-counter versions. Nonprescription NSAIDs include aspirin, ibuprofen, naproxen, and ketoprofen. About 20 percent of people who take NSAIDs regularly develop ulcers.
- Smoking, which increases the concentration and volume of acid in the stomach. Studies have found that smokers run a greater risk of developing ulcers.
- Excessive use of alcohol, which can erode the mucous lining in the stomach and intestines, causing inflammation. In this compromised state, the body is more vulnerable to invasion with *H. pylori* and other irritants.

If you have symptoms of an ulcer, consult your doctor for diagnosis and treatment.

Conclusion

Most of the patients who come to me for help with IBS have spent years going from one doctor to another, trying one medication after another. Each time, the treatment has failed, leaving the patient a bit more dispirited and a bit more doubtful of ever finding a cure. These cycles of hope and eventual failure can be emotionally challenging, often leading patients to blame themselves and wonder what they are doing to cause their problems to persist.

You need to remember that you are not alone in your suffering with IBS; millions of other people share your discomfort. More importantly, you must remember that you *can* live without digestive pain. By following the IBS Program I have presented here, you finally will be able to eliminate your IBS symptoms and become pain-free without dependence on over-the-counter medications or prescription drugs. Unlike other treatments for IBS, which tend to suppress the symptoms, I believe that you must look at your body holistically and deal with the cause of your gastrointestinal problems.

While most of my patients begin to feel better within days of starting the program, I urge you to be patient. You may have been suffering with IBS for months or years, and it may take several weeks or months to regain your overall health. You will have good days and bad days as you perform the detective work necessary to identify the foods that you need to eliminate from your diet. It can be time consuming and challenging to monitor your food intake and analyze your reactions to various foods, but this investment in time and energy will pay off with a lifetime eating plan that will help you regain balance in your digestive system.

I have made every attempt to present the information in this book in the same way that I would if you were a patient visiting my office. I have explained the various tests used to analyze your digestive health and to identify possible food hypersensitivities, and I have outlined a program of vitamin and nutritional supplement therapy to improve your gastrointestinal balance. Of course, every situation is different and every body faces unique challenges. If your IBS symptoms continue after following the advice in the book or if you have questions about the IBS treatment program, feel free to contact my medical practice at:

The Ash Center for Comprehensive Medicine
800A Fifth Avenue
New York, NY 10021-7216
(212) 758-3200
www.ashcenter.com

In addition, you can learn more about IBS and other health topics by tuning in to my radio talk show on Sunday from 5 to 7 P.M. on WOR-AM (710 AM) in New York. If you live outside the New York area, you can hear a live broadcast anywhere in the world during the same hours at www.alternativemedicineandhealth.com.

Resources

American Academy of Environmental Medicine
7701 East Kellogg, Suite 625
Wichita, KS 67207
(316) 684-5500
www.aaem.com

This academy strives to support physicians and other health care professionals through education about the interaction between people and their environment. The group sponsors conferences and training for health care professionals and the general public, and it publishes and distributes books, monographs, and audiotapes on environmental health subjects. The designation of Fellow is awarded to members who have successfully completed the Core Curriculum and passed the board examination of the American Board of Environment Medicine. The group also provides referrals to member physicians who have completed the academy's Core Curriculum.

American Association of Naturopathic Physicians
3201 New Mexico Avenue, NW
Suite 350
Washington, DC 20016
(866) 538-2267; (202) 895-1392
www.naturopathic.org

This association is a professional organization for naturopathic physicians. Naturopathic medicine focuses on whole-patient wellness, with an emphasis on prevention and self-care. The association publishes and distributes materials on a wide range of health topics.

American College of Advancement in Medicine (ACAM)
23121 Verdugo Drive, Suite 204
Laguna Hills, CA 92653
(949) 583-7666
www.acam.org

ACAM is a not-for-profit medical society dedicated to educating physicians and other health care professionals on preventive and nutritional medicine.

American Holistic Medical Association (AHMA)
12101 Menaul Boulevard Northeast
Suite C
Albuquerque, NM 87112
(505) 292-7788
www.holisticmedicine.org

The AHMA is a professional organization of licensed medical doctors (M.D.s) and doctors of osteopathic medicine (D.O.s) from every specialty who practice holistic medicine. Member physicians strive to address the physical, environmental, mental, emotional, spiritual, and social health of their patients. The association provides both a printed and an online directory of holistic physicians accepting referrals.

The Ash Center for Comprehensive Medicine

800A Fifth Avenue (61st Street)
New York, NY 10021-7216
(212) 758-3200
www.ashcenter.com

The Ash Center provides comprehensive treatment and prevention programs, including gastric analysis, nutritional counseling, vitamin supplement therapy, intravenous vitamin therapy, chelation allergy assessment and neutralization, and stress management, among others. Dr. Ash presents a radio talk show on Sunday from 5 to 7 P.M. on WOR-AM (710 AM) in New York, with a live global broadcast at www.alternativemedicineandhealth.com.

Celiac Disease Foundation

13251 Ventura Boulevard, #1
Studio City, CA 91604
(818) 990-2354
www.celiac.org

The Celiac Disease Foundation provides support, information, and assistance to people with celiac disease and dermatitis herpetiformis. It also sponsors a bulletin board and links to Web sites of interest.

Celiac Sprue Association/USA Inc.
P.O. Box 31700
Omaha, NE 68131-0700
(402) 558-0600
www.csaceliacs.org

This organization is dedicated to providing information and assistance to people with celiac disease and their families. The Web site includes recipes and product information for people who must eat a gluten-free diet.

Crohn's and Colitis Foundation of America
386 Park Avenue South
17th Floor
New York, NY 10016-8804
(800) 932-2423; (212) 685-3440
www.ccfa.org

This foundation strives to improve the quality of life for people suffering from Crohn's disease and colitis through education and support. It also provides updates on research, links to clinical trials, educational brochures, and information on finding a doctor with expertise in treating the conditions. The foundation sponsors chapters and local groups nationwide.

Digestive Disease National Coalition (DDNC)
507 Capitol Court, NE
Suite 200
Washington, DC 20002
(202) 544-7497
www.ddnc.org

This advocacy organization comprises several national societies concerned with digestive diseases. The DDNC focuses on increasing public awareness and improving public policy related to digestive diseases.

Gluten Intolerance Group of North America
15110 10th Avenue Southwest
Suite A
Seattle, WA 98166-1820
(206) 246-6652
www.gluten.net

The Gluten Intolerance Group is a nonprofit organization dedicated to increasing awareness of celiac disease and dermatitis herpetiformis. The group publishes a quarterly newsletter, distributes educational materials, sponsors lectures and meetings, and advocates on behalf of people with gluten intolerance. The group offers restaurant card tips with information to help people dining out.

International College of Integrative Medicine (ICIM)
8189 Faussett Road
Fenton, MI 48430
(866) 464-5226
www.glccm.org

The International College of Integrative Medicine is a not-for-profit medical society focused on educating health care professionals about the latest research-supported techniques and holistic therapies. It also provides a venue for physicians to share information on various approaches that work in clinical practice.

International Foundation for Functional Gastrointestinal Disorders

P.O. Box 170864
Milwaukee, WI 53217-8076
(414) 964-1799; (888) 964-2001
www.iffgd.org

This foundation is a nonprofit education and research organization dedicated to informing, assisting, and supporting people with gastrointestinal disorders, including IBS. The group also advocates for research funding through the National Institutes of Health.

National Cancer Institute

Public Inquiries Office
Building 31, Room 10A03
31 Center Drive, MSC 2580
Bethesda, MD 20892-2590
(800) 4-CANCER
www.cancernet.nci.nih.gov

The National Cancer Institute provides extensive information about all types of cancer, including cancers of the gastrointestinal tract.

National Digestive Diseases Information Clearinghouse

2 Information Way
Bethesda, MD 20892-3570
(310) 654-3810; (800) 891-5389
www.niddk.nih.gov/health/digest/nddic.htm

This clearinghouse is an information-dissemination service of the National Institute of Diabetes and Digestive and Kidney Diseases, which is part of the National Institutes of Health. The clearinghouse answers queries about digestive disease by phone (8:30 A.M. to 5 P.M. eastern standard time), fax, mail, and e-mail. It also provides a range of publications on various topics, including irritable bowel syndrome.

Pure Essentials® for Pharmaceutical Quality Vitamins
800 Fifth Avenue
New York, NY 10021
(800) 628-3009
http://alternativemedicineandhealth.com/vitamins/PE-overview.htm

Pure Essentials offers a product line of nutritional supplements.

ON THE WEB

Most of the Web sites listed above include links to chat rooms and informational sites for people with IBS.

- The Irritable Bowel Syndrome Page (www.healingwell.com/ibs) includes an IBS Resource Center with links to organizations, support groups, chat rooms, and research about IBS.
- The Irritable Bowel Syndrome Self Help and Support Group (www.ibsgroup.org) provides bulletin boards, studies, lists of medications, and general information about IBS.

Index

abdominal roll, 138
abdominal windmill, 139
acid-alkaline balance, 120
  of the body, 18–19
  of the gastrointestinal system, *see* pH of the gastrointestinal tract
acidophilus, 156–57
adrenaline, 119
aerobic exercise, 140–45
alcoholic beverages, 67, 92, 203–204, 214, 220
alkaline foods, accentuating, 76, 77
Alosetron (lotronex), 22
amaranth, 99
American Board of Hypnotherapy, 131
American Council of Hypnotist Examiners, 132
American Journal of Clinical Nutrition, 58, 60–61
American Massage Therapy Association, 134
American Oriental Bodywork Therapy Association, 134
American Society of Clinical Hypnosis, 132
amino acid complex, 158–59
antacids, 1, 2, 5–6, 7, 26, 65–66
antibiotics, 60, 67, 91
antibody response to foods, tests measuring, 7, 28–30, 47–48
antidepressants, 22–23
antidiarrheals, 21
antifungal medications, 71
antigens, 46
antispasmodic drugs, 22
anus, 16
Apple(s):
  Chutney with Brown Rice, 103
  Waldorf Salad, Breakfast, 105
Artichoke Hearts and Vegetables, Millet with, 110–11
Ash Center for Comprehensive Medicine, xiii, 222
Associated Bodywork and Massage Professionals, 134

Association for Applied Psychophysiology and Biofeedback, The, 130
avocado for Guacamole with Fresh Veggies, 110

Barrett's esophagus, 215
basal metabolic rate, 145, 147
basil for Pesto, 112
bile, 14
biofeedback, 129–30
biological terrain assessment, 26–28
birth control pills, 67
Black-Eyes Peas, Greens, and Millet, 104
blood chemistry test, 31
blood pressure, 141
B lymphocyte cells, 46
Board for Therapeutic Massage and Bodywork, 133
bovine growth hormone (rBGH), 60
breads, banishing (and other yeasty foods), 76, 77, 98
breakfast, *see* IBS Eating Plan; meal plans
Breakfast Broccoli with Brown Rice, 104–105
Breakfast Waldorf Salad, 105
breathing, deep, 122–24
Broccoli with Rice, Breakfast, 104–105
Brown Rice:
 Apple Chutney with, 103
 Breakfast Broccoli with, 104–105
buckwheat, 99
butter, 83
 Ghee-"Liquid Gold," 109–10

caffeine, 2
calcium, nondairy sources of, 57–59
Cambridge Insight Meditation Center, 126
cancer, 32, 137, 210–12
Candida albicans, 19, 64, 70
candidiasis, *see* yeast overgrowth
Cannon, Walter B., 118
carbohydrates:
 complex, low-sugar, 77
 simple, 68, 77
causes of IBS, 17–18, 117–18
celiac disease (gluten intolerance), 195–206
 cookbooks, gluten-free, 205
 diagnosing, 199–200
 eating out with, 204–205
 flour substitutes, gluten-free, 206
 foods you can and cannot eat, 201–202
 gluten-free diet, 198, 200–206
 the gluten response, 197–98
 reading food labels, 202–203
 risk factors, 196–97
 support groups, 201
 symptoms of, 196
Cereal with Fruit, Rise 'N' Shine, 113–14
chemical additives, eliminating foods with, 91–92, 98
chewing food, 90
child's pose, 139
cholesterol, 14, 94, 137
cobra pose, 139
colitis, 209–10
colon (large intestine), 15, 120
 X-ray (barium enema), 33–34
colon cancer, 210–12
colonoscopy, 36–37, 211–12
colon transit test, 39
colorectal cancer, 32, 211
complete blood count (CBC), 31
comprehensive stool test, 30
computed tomography (CT scan), 34–35, 213

condiments, 89–90
conventional vs. natural medicine, 40–41
cookbooks:
  dairy-free, 62
  gluten-free, 205
cortisol, 119
Crohn's disease, 208–209
Cucumber:
  Salad, 107
  Soup, Cold, 106

daily plan, thirty day, xiv–xv, 166–94
dairy products:
  Core Diet, 83
  eliminating, 76, 78, 98
  lactose intolerance, xiv, 54–63, 78
  other calcium sources, 57–59
  sensitivity to, 1–2, 18
  substitutes for, 61–63
dermatitis herpetiformis, 199
diagnosing celiac disease, 199–200
diagnosing IBS, 24–40
  finding the cause, 20
  tests for, *see* diagnostic tests
  traditional approach to, 6–7, 19–20
diagnostic tests, 20, 25–40
  measuring antibody response to foods, 7, 28–30, 47–48
diet:
  elimination, 29, 49–50
  gluten-free, for celiac disease, 198, 200–206
  IBS Eating Plan, *see* IBS Eating Plan
  yeast overgrowth treated with, 71–74
digestive process, explanation of, 9–16
dinner, *see* IBS Eating Plan; meal plans
diverticulitis and diverticulosis, 212–13
doctors:
  consulting, 149, 166
  finding the right, 40–42
  questions to ask prospective, 43
duodenum, 13, 14

eating out with celiac disease, 204–205
Eggplant:
  Ratatouille, 112–13
  Salad, Chilled, 105–106
elimination diet, 29, 49–50
ELISA/ACT (enzyme-linked immunosorbent assay) test, 29–30
emotional stress, xiv, 7, 117–18
  see also stress
endoscopy, 35–37
epinephrine, 119
esophagus, 11, 213–14, 215
  cancer of the, 210
essential fatty acids, 90, 94–95
exercise, xiv, 136–61
  aerobic fitness, 140–45
  benefits of, 137–38
  daily plans, 166–94
  in daily routine, 149–50
  for flexibility, 147–48
  getting started, 148–49
  intestinal exercises, 138–39
  strength training, 145–46
  warm up and cool down, 143

family practice doctors, 41
fats, dietary, 94–95
  Core Diet, 90
fiber supplements, 21
fight-or-flight response, 118–19
fish, 82, 95
flatus, 15
flexibility, 147–48
food allergies, xiv, 6, 18, 19, 45–54, 120, 157
  common allergenic foods, 50
  delayed, symptoms of, 50–51

eliminating and reintroducing foods, 53–54
identifying, on your own, 49–52
leaky gut syndrome and, 53–54
testing for, 8, 28–30, 47–48, 52
Food and Drug Administration, 164–65
food diary, 50, 79
daily plan, 168–94
food sensitivities, xiv, 2, 6, 18, 45–54
testing for, 8, 28–30
Foundation of Human Understanding, 126, 127
fowl, 82, 91
fruits, 91
Cereal with, Rise 'N' Shine, 113–14
Core Diet, 87–89
Salad, 107

gallbladder, 14, 35
cancer of the, 211
Garbanzo Spread, 107–108
gastric analysis test (Heidelberg test), 25–26
gastric emptying, 38
and small-bowel transit, 38
gastroenterologists, 40
Gastroenterology Nursing, 136
gastroesophageal reflux disease (GERD), 213–15
gastrointestinal tract:
functions of, 3
pH of, *see* pH of the gastrointestinal tract
Gazpacho, 108
general practitioners, 42
Ghee-"Liquid Gold," 109–10
Gi Gong, 135–36
ginger tea, 161–62
glucagons, 13
glucose, 14, 68
glutamine, 155–56
gluten intolerance, *see* celiac disease (gluten intolerance)
grains, 86–87, 99–100
Cereal with Fruit, Rise 'N' Shine, 113–14
see also specific grains
Guacamole with Fresh Veggies, 110

heartburn, 143, 213, 215
heart rate, target, 141–42
Helicobacter pylori, 26, 65, 219–20
high-density lipoprotein (HDL) cholesterol, 94
holistic approach to treating IBS, 4
overview, ix, xii, xiii–xv
see also specific measures, e.g. exercise; IBS Eating Plan
hydrochloric acid, 5, 12–13, 65, 120
hypnosis, 130–32

IBS Eating Plan, xiv, 19, 75–96
core principles of, 76–78
daily plans, 166–94
foods to choose for Core Diet, 81–90
general guidelines for healthy eating, 90–93
phase 1: healing and repair with core foods, 78–79, 100–101
phase 2: reintroducing foods one at a time, 80, 102–103
phase 3: maintenance (lifetime), 80–81, 102–103
preparing your kitchen, 98
recipes, 103–16
time-saving tips, 100
ileum, 14
immune system response, 46–47
immunosuppressant drugs, 67
inflammatory bowel disease (IBD), 209
insulin, 13

Internal Yoga Institute, 136
internists, 42
intestinal hand massage, 138–39

jejunum, 14
Journal of Clinical Psychiatry, 117

kitchen, preparing your, 98

labels, reading food, 92, 202–203
lactase, 57
lactose intolerance, xiv, 54–63, 78
large intestine, *see* colon (large intestine)
laxatives, 21
leaky gut syndrome, 53–54, 119, 120
liquid-only diet, 79, 92–94
liver (organ), 13–14, 35, 94, 158
  cancer of the, 211
lunch, *see* IBS Eating Plan; meal plans
lymphatic system, benefits of exercise for, 144–45

magnesium, 57, 59, 119
massage, 132–34
meal plans:
  phase 1, 100–101
  phase 2 and 3, 102–103
meals, eating three balanced, 91
meats, 82–83, 91
medications:
  masking of symptoms with, x, 20
  over-the-counter, *see* over-the-counter medications
  prescription, *see* prescription drugs
meditation, 124–27
milk intolerance, *see* lactose intolerance
millet, 99
  with Artichoke Hearts and Vegetables, 110–11
  Black-Eyed Peas, Greens, and, 104
  Wraps, Vegetable Salad, 115–16
Mind/Body Medical Institute, The, 126
minerals and other nutritional supplements, xiv, 57, 152–65
Minestrone, 111–12
monounsaturated fats, 95
multivitamins, 159–61

National Certification Board of Therapeutic Massage, 133
National Guild of Hypnotists, 132
natural medicine, 40–41
naturopathic physicians, 42
nonsteroidal antiinflammatory drugs (NSAIDs), 220
Nurses Health Study, Harvard University, 61
nursing mothers, 70
nut milk, homemade, 63
nutritional supplements, xiv, 19, 152–65
  choosing the right brand, 164–65
  daily plans, 166–94
  phase 1, 153–57
  phase 2, 158–64
  troubleshooting, 158
nuts and seeds, 83–84

omega-3 and omega-6 fatty acids, 95
organic foods, 79, 91
osteoporosis, 59
overeating, 91
over-the-counter medications, 1, 4, 20–21

pancreas, 13, 35, 66, 120
  cancer of the, 211
pancreatitis, 216–17
parasites, 217–18
parotid glands, 10

peptic ulcers, 218–20
pesticides, 25, 47, 60, 91
Pesto, 112
pH of the gastrointestinal tract, xiii, 2, 5–6, 18–19, 66, 157
physicians, *see* doctors
polyunsaturated fats, 95
poultry, 82, 91
prescription drugs, 1, 4, 5, 7, 21–23, 26, 71
  antacids, 1, 2, 5–6, 7, 26, 65–66
  antibiotics, 60, 67
  antifungals, 71
  GERD and, 215
  side effects of, 6
prevention, xv
processed foods, 79, 98
progressive relaxation, 127
prostate cancer, 60–61
protein, 77
pulse rate, target, 141–42
pyloric valve, 13

Qi Gong, 135–36
quercetin, 155
quinoa, 99–100
  Cereal with Fruit, Rise 'N' Shine, 113–14

radiological procedures, 32–40
RAST test (radioallergosorbent test), 28–29, 30
Ratatouille, 112–13
recipes, 103–16
relaxation techniques, 122–35
  daily plans, 167–94
resources, 223–29
Royal Free Hospital, London, 130

Salad:
  Cucumber, 107
  Eggplant, Chilled, 105–106
  Fruit, 107
  Turkey and Vegetable, 114–15
  Waldorf, Breakfast, 105
salivary glands, 10–11
salt, 91
saturated fats, 94, 95
sauna, 150–51
seeds and nuts, 83–84
shellfish, 82
sigmoidoscopy, 37
small intestine, 13–14, 120
  cancer of the, 210
  X-ray, 33
smoking, 149, 214, 220
snacks, 91
  phase 1, 101
soft drinks, 98
Soup:
  Cucumber, Cold, 106
  Gazpacho, 108
  Minestrone, 111–12
sphincter muscle, 16, 214–15, 215
Steam-Fry, Vegetable, 116
stomach, 120, 214
  cancer of the, 210
  digestive process in the, 12–13
stomach flapping, 138
stool, 15
  comprehensive stool test, 30, 70
  hemoccult test, 32
  parasite test, 32
strength training, 145–46
stress, 17
  emotional, *see* emotional stress
  physiology of, 118–21
  relaxation techniques, 122–35
  types of, 121
stretching, 147–48
String Beans Vinaigrette, 114
sublingual glands, 10–11

submandibular glands, 10
sugar, 2, 67, 71, 77, 98
supplements, *see* nutritional supplements
symptoms of celiac disease, 196
symptoms of IBS, 3, 16–17
  resembling problems of other digestive disorders, xv, 17, 24, 30, 207–208

target heart rate, 141–42
teas, 93, 94, 161–62
teff, 100
thirty-day plan to a healthier digestive system, 166–94
traditional approach to treatment of IBS:
  problems with, 5–7
Transcendental Meditation, 124
trans-fatty acids, 94, 95, 98
transit studies, 38–40
Turkey and Vegetable Salad, 114–15

ulcerative colitis, 209–10
ultrasound, 35
University of North Carolina, 130
upper endoscopy (esophagogastroduodenoscopy, or EGD), 36
urine tests, 31

vegetables, 91
  calcium from leafy green, 57, 58
  Core Diet, 84–86
  Guacamole with Fresh, 110
  Millet with Artichoke Hearts and, 110–11
  Salad Wraps, 115–16
  Steam-Fry, 116
  Turkey and, Salad, 114–15
  see also specific vegetables
vinegars, gluten-free diet and, 203–204
visualization, 127–28
vitamin C, 154–55, 163–64
vitamin D, 57
vitamins and other nutritional supplements, xiv, 6, 152–65

Waldorf Salad, Breakfast, 105
walking, 143, 144
water, 90–91, 93
whole-gut transit test, 39
Wraps, Vegetable Salad, 115–16

yeast, eliminating dietary, 77
yeast overgrowth, xiv, 1, 18, 19, 64–74
  development of, 65–67
  symptoms of, 68–70
  treatment with diet, 71–74
yoga, 134–35

Zelnorm, 21–22
Zollinger-Ellison syndrome, 214–15